Julie Sceeny is an i̶   and teacher trainer. She has been teaching for many years, she has taught over 15000 classes and run more than 25 teacher-training courses. Other than teaching, her passion is training and educating people to become teachers, seeing people grow and change. Julie has taught in Europe and Asia for many years and has gained a wealth of knowledge, of the skill of teaching which she always likes to pass onto fellow teachers. Teaching is not the same as it was years ago and so Julie likes to keep updated on new terms and ideas around the best way to teach.

This book is dedicated to everyone that has come into my life. Good or bad, you have taught me a lesson which brings me to the point I am at now. Without taking the journey I have, I would not be where I am now, so I am grateful for that.

Julie Sceeny

CHANGE

A Book for Yoga Teachers

AUSTIN MACAULEY PUBLISHERS™
LONDON • CAMBRIDGE • NEW YORK • SHARJAH

Copyright © Julie Sceeny 2024

The right of Julie Sceeny to be identified as author of this work has been asserted by the author in accordance with sections 77 and 78 of the Copyright, Designs and Patents Act 1988.

All rights reserved. No part of this publication may be reproduced, stored in a retrieval system, or transmitted in any form or by any means, electronic, mechanical, photocopying, recording, or otherwise, without the prior permission of the publishers.

Any person who commits any unauthorised act in relation to this publication may be liable to criminal prosecution and civil claims for damages.

The story, experiences, and words are the author's alone.

A CIP catalogue record for this title is available from the British Library.

ISBN 9781398494572 (Paperback)
ISBN 9781398494589 (ePub e-book)

www.austinmacauley.com

First Published 2024
Austin Macauley Publishers Ltd®
1 Canada Square
Canary Wharf
London
E14 5AA

I want to say a huge thanks to Justin and Flynn, my dear friends and my amazing models. Justin, thanks for always believing in me and pushing me, you helped me believe in myself, much love.

Thank you to those that have continued to support me through this magical journey called life.

Table of Contents

Chapter 1: Opening   **16**

Why this book?   *16*

Yoga teacher training   *20*

Feedback and lessons during my teaching journey   *25*

Yoga, Thailand, and me   *32*

Chapter 2: Role of the Teacher   **39**

The role of the teacher   *40*

Your favourite teacher versus your least favourite   *45*

How to teach a yoga class   *49*

After teacher training   *51*

Chapter 3: Understanding Poses   **57**

Understanding yoga poses   *57*

Why are some poses difficult or easy for some people?   *58*

Knowing modifications   *61*

Downward Dog   *62*

Downward Dog   *67*

So what are the benefits of a Downward Dog?	73
How do you know if it is muscle tightness or something else?	73
How to modify Downward Dog	76
Mobility, stability and flexibility	76
Chapter 4: Dialogue	**78**
Verbal instructions	78
So why does it matter what we say?	80
Person or pose set up dialogue	82
In posture dialogue	82
Exit dialogue	83
Power words vs. powerless words	84
Powerless words – Examples	84
Power words – Examples	85
Types of cues	86
General dialogue	87
Lock your (knees/elbows)	89
Awkward pose	94
Feet hips distance apart	96
Feet parallel	97
Arms up	99
Sit down	101
Pelvis	102

Possible Cues:	*105*
Hips flexed – What muscles flex the hips	*115*
Knees flexed	*116*
Feet hips distance apart	*116*
Shoulders are flexed and internally rotated	*116*
Ankles dorsiflexed	*116*
How to give corrective cues	*118*
Chapter 5: Voice	**120**
Why is the voice so important?	*120*
Tone of voice	*121*
Examples of different tones	*121*
Change your tone for certain parts for the class	*124*
Exiting a pose	*124*
Change your tone for certain classes	*125*
Chapter 6: Body Language	**126**
Your own body language whilst teaching	*126*
Hands on hips	*127*
Clasping hands in the front	*128*
Checking out the nails	*129*
Chapter 7: Demonstration of Poses	**131**
Should we demonstrate poses in class?	*131*
How do we teach poses we can't actually do?	*131*
How much of class should we practise with students?	*132*

Chapter 8: Room Position 134

Where is it appropriate to stand?   134

Understand personal space   136

How to move around the room   137

Chapter 9: Adjustments 138

Should we offer adjustments in class?   138

How to adjust students   139

Know your students   141

Injuries   145

Chapter 10: Class Structure 148

Basic class structure   148

Mistakes often made by new teachers   151

How to structure a class?   156

Reverse engineering – Bird of paradise   159

Factors to consider when structuring a class   162

How long is the warm-up and cool-down?   163

Do we include meditation?   163

Does the day of the week matter?   169

How about different times of the year or seasons?   170

Seasons   170

Chapter 11: Breathing Exercises/Pranayama 171

Benefits of breathing exercises   171

½ Litre V 3.5 Litres   173

So what are the benefits of deep breathing? 174

How do you use the full lung capacity? 174

What can restrict us? 174

Benefits of deep breathing 175

Examples of breathing exercises 176

Kapalbhati – mouth or nose version (breath of fire) 178

Inhale and exhale for four counts 179

Alternate nostril breathing 180

Chapter 12: Meditation **183**

Benefits of meditation 183

How to teach meditation 184

Examples of mediation – Prep, finisher and samples 184

Golden Bay 187

Behind the Falls 189

The Rocking Chair 191

The orchard 192

Chapter 13: Teaching Online **196**

How to teach online 196

Interaction with students 202

Mistakes made by most teachers 203

Style of yoga classes you can teach online 203

Conclusion **205**

"An investment in knowledge pays the best interest."
– Benjamin Franklin

Chapter 1
Opening

Why this book?

It's April 2020 and the world is in lockdown due to COVID-19. My name is Julie and I'm a yoga and pilates teacher. I live and work in Bangkok and having spent two and a half months in the UK taking care of my dying mother. I returned to Thailand to find things not quite the same: studios are closed, shops are closed, and people are encouraged to work from home. However, there aren't any restrictions on moving around during the daytime other than wearing a facemask and maintaining social distance. Although not everyone has been able to work during this pandemic, as the head teacher at the studio where I've worked for 10 years, I kept busy most days helping film live online yoga and pilates classes.

One of my roles as head teacher is teacher training, so with all studios closed, this was the perfect time to hold workshops and trainings for our teachers. It was an interesting time and to be honest; it worked for me. My life is always hectic and busy, and I never get around to doing things I want to do outside of work, like writing this book. Working less allowed me to slow down and reflect, and so my goal here is to share my knowledge about teaching to help others improve their own teaching and yoga practice.

The world as we know it might not be exactly the same again and training courses will certainly move online so this is a good time to share with a wider community all that I've learned over many years of teaching and training. Teaching online is a new experience for most but it combines two of my passions, teaching yoga and working in the film industry. One thing I've realised is that teaching online requires different skills, better dialogue and cues, and a different way of teaching, which ultimately led to this book. This book is not designed to just be able to teach online, but also how to improve your teaching so that when life is more 'normal,' we can be much better teachers. I hope you enjoy this journey and that if you only learn but one thing, it will have been worthwhile to read this guide.

First, thank you for buying this book, for showing you care about your job and teaching so much that you want to improve yourself. It's easy to become complacent, especially if you've been teaching for a few years. Once we get too familiar with a job, it's easy to skip the planning and preparation and just show up to teach. If you want to plod along and earn some coins while doing an adequate job, that's perfectly fine. However, if you want to become the best teacher, you can be and keep your skills sharp, you have to improve yourself by studying or taking courses.

Fresh-faced teachers come along all the time, and studios will get rid of deadweight if they find new people coming along with a passion to learn who can also teach a great class.

The fact that you bought this book shows you're keen to learn and that puts you on the path to being a better teacher in itself. You made a decision at some point to become a yoga teacher and now you're taking the next step, which is to improve yourself. This book found you to help you become a better teacher, so I promise you that if you learn the tips and tricks I offer in this book, then you will become a better teacher. By reading this book, I hope to make your journey a quicker one to becoming the best teacher you can be. I've detailed and condensed years of work and practice into a book that you can carry with you on your journey as a yoga teacher. You might not be able to apply everything all at once, but take one part each week and focus on that until it's second-nature and then take one more point and within a few months, you'll see change.

I don't have all the answers, but I do have well-honed ideas about the best way to teach as everything I write about in this book I've taught to hundreds of teachers worldwide and the results speak for themselves. I've been to many yoga classes all over the world and have experienced different teachers and different yoga styles. During the majority of classes, I ended up spending time during the class thinking about how the teacher could improve their own teaching. Of course, I've been to some amazing classes, but they are few and far between. Obviously, this is just my opinion as to what and how I think a teacher should teach, but it's based on a vast amount of experience in both teaching classes and training teachers.

When you first go to class, you may not know how long the teacher has been teaching, but you'll decide if you like the class and/or the teacher right away, so it's important to do your best and keep studying and learning to improve. The tricky thing as a new teacher is that the best way to get better at teaching is to teach and teach a lot, meaning definitely teaching some tough classes, which is normal as long as you're humble and remember that we're in the service industry and you remember the expectations.

When you go into a coffee shop, what do you expect from the staff? They may not make the perfect coffee, especially if they're new, but if they're super friendly and nice you might forgive them. Someone giving you a big smile when you're having a bad day can make all the difference in how you feel the rest of the day. If they're a little rude and maybe not so friendly, but they make the perfect coffee will you forgive them? It's all down to expectations. No one teacher can deliver the perfect class that satisfies everyone at all times but we can be humble and keep trying. Imagine if you go to an early morning class before work the effect of that class can affect your whole day. If the teacher was late, rude, and very strict, you might leave in a more aggressive mood, which you then take with you on your day. Verses a super nice class where the teacher was friendly, they also complimented you on a pose and you left feeling great. This class has set you up for your workday and can determine what mood you are in. Which yes, of course, the same thing could happen in a coffee shop too. Imagine if you could have affected someone so that they leave feeling good, they are nice to everyone at work. They are nice to the coffee shop barista, they get through the day's work without drama and they go home feeling good and finish the day with a good feeling. So many people can be affected by the result of that one yoga class. Maybe a little dramatic, possibly but what we do does affect how people feel and our job is to make them feel better than when they came in. Of course, I don't expect everyone to be amazing, good is enough but I have been to many below-average classes. Or to classes where the teacher is over confident, they know it all and certainly would not be open to receiving feedback.

So who am I and why do I think I am qualified to write this book well, that comes a little later…

Yoga teacher training

As I said previously some teacher's classes I experienced were not that great. Even though I say a teacher was average, this is possibly not their fault, they are possibly teaching the way they were trained to teach. So they don't know any different, they simply teach the way they were shown. It's only when they take further courses or training and learn from others that they begin to change. I am not suggesting that the teacher trainer is bad, either people tend to teach the way they know and often it works, what I am offering is a method that gives you all the skills to become a great teacher.

It's all too easy to take a short course online and become a teacher, without having actually taught any physical students. It's like asking a chef to send a picture of his omelette without you actually tasting it. Omelettes are not easy and in order to perfect an omelette, you need to cook many omelettes. Much like teaching yoga the best way to improve is to teach. I see quite often that someone attends a training course and after a couple of years of teaching they decide they need something more so they set up and run their own teacher training course. I am not saying that is wrong but how do you know when you are ready to become a teacher trainer? It's a huge responsibility to train people to become good instructors and requires years of experience and knowledge.

I am not suggesting there is only one way to teach and that's it follow the rules, but the method I use has worked for many years and has helped me train hundreds of students who are now successful yoga teachers. I know many teachers who don't follow all of the suggestions I put in the book, but that does not make them bad teachers. In fact, I know some who can fill classes. It can take years to get to that point so I am helping you to get there just that little but quicker. A yoga class is an experience, so make it a good experience.

Yoga, as we know, comes from India years ago and even now people go to India to study yoga. However, the process of study is different from the west, in India, you find a guru and you practise with that guru. The focus initially is on practice, understanding your body and moving through the sequence. Once you have chosen a guru, you tend to stick with that method of learning and stay with that Guru. Some of the most obvious choices years ago would have been Iyengar or Pattabhi Jois. Each year, students go to India to study for 2–3 months at a time. The focus is on the practice and then maybe study philosophy and history such as the Vedas, Upanishads, Sutras and Bhagavad Gita. Each year you make the same trip and each year the guru assesses how well you are doing with the practice and study. The next stage would be assisting in classes and maybe then teaching.

For ashtanga yoga, you need to learn the count and the Sanskrit names plus transitions. The guru will decide when you are ready to teach and, although there might not be a formal exam as such, there are other criteria that determine when you are ready. For the most part, the focus is on the practice and how you are dedicated to that. This, of course, does not work for everyone, as taking that much time away from life can be tricky, work, family, etc. are real-life commitments that can't just be dropped every year for three months. Which is why a one-month training course in Bali is much more feasible than 2–3 months per year travelling to India. One month in Bali, you get your certificate and off you go. With the traditional Indian method, the guru determines if you are ready to teach. In the west, a 200-hour teaching certificate and maybe a yoga alliance membership determines you are okay to teach.

So which method is better? Can the guru in India make a better decision than the teacher trainer in Bali? Who knows? The focus in India seems to be on practice and getting that engrained in your body, which is not a bad thing, however teaching is a different concept. Neither is right nor wrong; they are just different.

So how do you feel about your teaching, do you think there is anything that can be improved? I have been teaching for 17 years and I still think I can improve; there is always more to learn. Think about the first class you ever taught, what was your teaching like? Is it the same now? It shouldn't be. Every time you teach, it's a different experience from which you should learn something. It might be something small like a tone of voice change or a word you say. But refining your teaching should always be something you strive to achieve.

How much have you tried to improve yourself during the time you have been teaching?

Have you taken extra courses? What tends to happen with new teachers is comparison. Oh, I want to teach like Jane; she is so good. It is good to have a teacher you like and a style you enjoy but remember you are an individual; there is only one Jane so be the best of yourself.

Unless you have been through the exact same life path as Jane, you won't be the same. Students in my course would often say, "But I want to teach like you Julie or be like you."

I would tell them, "I have been doing this for 17 years. You have just started, you can't compare us as we are in different parts of our journey. My part 10 is different to your part 1 and when you get to part 10, it will still not be the same as mine."

So why did I become a teacher trainer? It's not something I just decided I wanted to do. I was asked to join the team and it seemed like the perfect chance to help change lives.

Even as a teacher and a teacher trainer, I am always a student, the more I know the more I realise I don't know and it makes me want to study harder. I wanted to become a teacher trainer so I could have an impact on so many people's lives. I also wanted to increase the standard of teachers, sending out teachers that are good makes me proud. Don't get me wrong I failed some people, if you were not good enough or you did not work hard enough for it, I would fail people as, I did not want to send out sub-standard teachers. I am sure if you are reading this you might not be thinking about becoming a teacher trainer but I wanted to give some background on me, and my thoughts on the matter so you know where I am coming from. I am also not just someone who thought, *Okay let's write a book and see what happens*. I have run short courses in studios all over the world and many times people have said I learned more here today than in my 200-hour teacher training course. Therefore it's my duty to share the information in order to help improve the quality of teaching worldwide.

The first training course I took was great, but in reality, we can't take it all in the first time around, it's all too much new information at once, hence I decided to write a book. The aim of this book is for teachers who have been teaching anything from six months to 20 years and who would like to refine their teaching. I have some great simple tips that can change the way you teach in a short period of time. I teach much of this during my training courses but the reality is, there is so much information to take in and that not everything can be consumed during the one-month training.

The other difference I noticed between yoga qualifications and pilates qualifications is that there is no requirement to continue to learn yoga in order to keep your qualification as there is with pilates. Each year, I am required to take a number of hours of pilates training in order to keep my certification valid. I believe as people who work with people's bodies, we should continue to learn and keep up to date. My yoga certification is valid for the rest of my life. Of course, if I don't clock up training hours I might not be able to register with certain yoga institutions but with my pilates qualification if I don't keep up my hours I will need to retake the exam (at a cost) to keep my qualification valid.

I always tell people that have attended my training course that actually the real learning starts when you leave the comfort of the course and you start teaching the general public. Normally at that point, the support network might not be there anymore and so you are alone. Then you must teach real students which is so much harder than your peers. In a real group class, there is much more of a mixed level of students, you might have some very experienced students and some brand-new students. Your job as a teacher is to ensure the experience is good for all. New students should not be scared and the experienced ones should leave feeling good.

Feedback and lessons during my teaching journey

The best way to improve as a teacher is to take courses, keep studying, and to ask for feedback. As new teachers, we often ask people for feedback but I have found more often that not only are people too afraid to give feedback, they sometimes don't know how to do it. If someone does not like a teacher, they will just never go to their class again. I know that because I have done the same thing, if I don't know that person and they don't ask for feedback I feel it's not my place to give it. Sometimes students don't know what it is they don't like about a class they just don't like the class; it could be a combination of things. This does not help a teacher to grow and learn as feedback helps you to improve and adjust your class according to the studio or group you are teaching. Feedback can come from students, fellow teachers or the people who work at the studio such as the studio manager. Of course, feedback will be someone's personal opinion, but you never know what you might learn from it. I still to this day, ask for feedback if teachers come to my class. Most of the time people don't give it but I ask because I believe if you are prepared to give feedback you should be prepared to receive it too.

For me, feedback is not about criticising someone, it's about giving them tools that they can use to improve their classes. You may or may not agree with what I suggest, but that's okay, I am just sharing my years of experience in the hope that you get at least one gem of information. The more I know the more I realise I don't know so I continually educate myself to try to improve so that I can pass on what I have learned.

It's true that after a few years some teachers can get bored or stale in terms of their teaching. Unless you are a creature of habit and you like to do the same thing every day, teaching at the same studio with the same people can get a little boring after 10 years. So how do you make teaching not boring or stale? How do you bring life back into teaching? For me, this has not been the case because I strive to be the best I can be and through education, I keep learning and improving. It is true if we say the same thing every day it can be boring so find new things to say, express yourself differently, learn why students can't do certain things, and examine how we can deliver the same information in another way to make it clear.

When I started teaching, I was no different to you but after many years, I have learnt many lessons, which I want to share in the hope you can learn them before you make the same mistakes I did when we first start teaching. We want to be great teachers and we are very sensitive to everything, the one thing that will be a constant on your mind is the following thought, *I am a bad teacher*. I want you to take that idea write it on a piece of paper and burn it.

We create thoughts in our head but they are not based on any evidence other than our own insecurities. It is normal when we start something new that we will be insecure and we can't expect to be perfect when we start; it takes time and effort. I believe we can achieve anything we want but we need to put in the effort. Achieving something through hard work is so much more satisfying too. The first time you cook a poached egg it generally goes wrong, well it did for me, but you keep trying and eventually you get better. It's fair to say though I am still rubbish at poaching eggs, but it's not something I care enough about so I don't practice enough but teaching is different.

You put the effort in to take a training course; training does not finish when the course finishes, it just begins. I like to think of the journey of teaching as the same as climbing a mountain. It's not easy; there are times when you will want to quit because it's too tough.

It's so much easier just to go back down the mountain, but if you equip yourself with the right tools you can make, the 'climb', easier. If you were to climb a mountain, you would need ropes, a harness, good shoes and an ice axe. So teaching what you need, some training aids such as books, videos, training courses and of course students. Your course should give you some knowledge but the students will teach you so much more.

The one thing that you are also not taught in many training courses is that practice teaching with your fellow trainees is easy. Teaching real students is a whole different game. Teaching teachers is easy because most of the time they know what to do and can follow instructions. Real people who maybe have not done much yoga or exercise per se are not used to moving in these ways and will not understand simple cues like feet parallel, or bend your elbow. I know that sounds crazy how can someone not know how to bend their elbow, trust me it's happened many times to me in the past. As a teacher is super daunting, when you look at some students and you see the position they are in and you think, *How do I fix that*, sometimes it's just best to ignore it because trying to fix it could mean you lose focus and if there is that much wrong they would need too much attention. I will discuss later how to deal with things like this that will come up in class.

For now, let's look at us as new teachers and the sort of things we say to ourselves when we first start teaching. The best way to get better at teaching is to actually teach but of course, there is a period of time when we are new teachers and during that time, each time we teach we get better. It is perfectly natural that some students will love your class and some won't like it. Even for me after over 17 years of teaching some people still might not like my class and that's okay. Because like students I also have certain preferences in terms of teachers I like and don't like. Of course, at first, I wanted everyone to love me and if people did not come to class it was because they did not like my class, or me this was not always the case, which I did not know at the time. When students don't come to class, we assume it's because of us, but in reality, life happens and people get busy.

Here are some ideas you may have had:

1. The students did not come to class because they did not like me.
2. I taught a bad class.
3. Is it because I forgot to do warrior 2 on the left side.
4. She/he hates me, her face says it all.
5. She/he walked out of class halfway through.

Let's examine each point:

1. Students did not come to class.

    - The reality is people get busy with life; the kids have parents' evening, people are too tired to come to class or there is a family dinner. Life takes over and sometimes they can't come to class. It's not always your class that is the issue.
    - It is also true that some won't like your style of teaching but that is okay. As long as you stay true to yourself and your character then you will find the right people that will connect with your class. Don't try to change to be something you are not to please people. Teaching comes from the heart and should be genuine to you.
    - When I first started teaching one week, I would have 10 people in class, the next it was three, I assumed it was me; I was a bad teacher, and I did something wrong.

2. Does it really matter if I forgot warrior 2?

    - Not really, it's not ideal but in the bigger picture, it's not a major mistake. Most of the time the students will know at the time that you forgot something but after class, they won't remember.

3. She/he hates me her face says it all.

    - 100% sure there will be a student in the class and they have what I call the 'bitch' face on. They hate you it's true, actually, it's not. I have been wrong on this so many times. I can tell that the woman in blue hates me and then after class, she comes up and says, "That was such an amazing class thanks so much." Some people are serious about their yoga and they practice with a serious look on their faces, they might not laugh at your jokes either but it does not mean they hate you. Hate is such a strong emotion anyway. I am not sure someone will ever feel that about a teacher, they might not like the class or connect with your personality but you would have to do a lot wrong even for someone to dislike you.

4. She/he walked out of class halfway through.

    - It happens and sometimes we don't know why. I have had women leave because they started their period or they need the bathroom. Maybe they are just not feeling it today or maybe they feel emotional. Yoga can bring up a lot of things for people and we don't know what is going on in someone's life that day so I say, always be kind. We often want to be so strict about being there on time and don't leave early etc. Of course, there are rules and guidelines that the studio might impose. But sometimes we just need to let some things go and not take them personally. They may be grieving, or they may have had a bad day at work, what we say and do in class can have a huge effect on someone's day. I personally like to think that I might have made someone's day easier or better or just made him or her feel good.

The things that we can control, outside of our teaching, are how we interact with students before and after class. Did you take any time to say hello, ask how they are or learn their name? I found these are some very simple things we can do to make students feel welcome. They will remember if you were nice to them, did you talk to them after or before class or if you complimented them for trying. Students will forgive a number of mistakes if they simply like the teacher because they are nice.

Many times, I have said left not right or almost forgot something but I am honest and am not afraid to admit I am human. I always say we are not heart surgeons if they make a mistake someone's life is in their hands, if we say left not right it does not matter that much. Not being able to do the perfect pose or admitting to a mistake makes us human. So what if you are having a bad day, or your cat just died or maybe you don't feel like it today. Maybe you're tired from teaching so many classes. My response is always the same, don't ever take anything you own into class. Students come to class for an experience. They don't need to know what is going on in your life, otherwise, suddenly the class is about you, the teacher and not the students. There are some teachers out there who put themselves on a pedestal and think the class should be about them. I believe as teachers we are simply guides, helping students through their practice. Much like your hiking guide will take you up the mountain, they will know the best route and the equipment to use. In the end, you actually have to climb the mountain. Yourself. The student needs to actually do the yoga; we just help facilitate them on their journey.

Every single class needs to be exactly the same and so you try your best. You give lots of energy and try not to let any of your emotions show. What you do and say will have an effect on their class and of course, we want them to go out feeling good. It's much like if you go into a bank and the teller is stroppy and aggressive, that does not make you feel good so don't offer the same treatment to your students. Then after class, go home and cry or do whatever you need to do but keep your problems your problems. I am not saying you can't talk to students; I am saying don't let any of your emotions or feelings affect how you teach. Be humble and kind and you will always have students, at the end of the day without students we don't have a job.

Yoga, Thailand, and me

I believe we can achieve anything we want as long as we want it badly enough. Of course, it needs to be a realistic goal and one that can be achieved, like running a marathon or losing weight, but wanting to be over six feet tall isn't realistic, as I stand here at a petite five-feet-one-inch tall.

If you have real passion, you can achieve anything even despite less-than-ideal external circumstances. I got to where I am now through passion and hard work and each part of my journey was a lesson. We learn from mistakes and times of trouble; happy times don't teach us as much as difficult times do. So, embrace the difficult times because if you overcome the challenges, the end goal feels like so much more.

If you look back at your own teacher training, it was probably hard work, physically, emotionally, and mentally. However, that moment at graduation when you knew you had done it and that all the hard work was worth it, is a feeling of immense joy. It wouldn't be the same if you were just handed a certificate without having done very much.

Dreams can be achieved despite obstacles in the way, which I believe present themselves to test if you really want to achieve a goal. Sometimes obstacles are also in the way to slow you down so that you are fully ready to become who you need to be when the time is right.

We are given lessons and sometimes we learn from them and sometimes we don't, and if we don't learn the first time, the same lesson will keep cropping up until we do. It's not always obvious at first what the lesson is, but when we're ready to learn, we will. I've had many difficult lessons over the past 50 years, but I wouldn't change anything because it made me who I am and has made life's journey worth it because the hard work does pay off in the end.

Why did you come to yoga? Why did you decide to become a yoga teacher? It is important to know why you are here? So take a moment to think about that. Take some time to think about what brought you here, the life journey you have taken so far. It's not always obvious at first but given time it will become clearer. I had a student come to one of my training courses and in week two she seriously hurt her knee so much that she could not practice, she was super frustrated as she had to sit on a mat during class whilst everyone else practised. I know what you are thinking, why attend class if you can't practice, you can still hear the dialogue and take time to learn the sequence. Observing classes can be a great way to learn many skills about teaching which you don't often see when you are practising.

So for this one student, there were many tears during this time, she was super emotional due to the frustration of not being able to practice. Of course, we all learn after the lesson and now she knows it was the best thing to happen. She learned about pushing too hard about doing things wrong and what effect it has on your body. The injury was pre-existing the two classes per day just brought the issue to the surface. She is now a very good teacher and her focus when teaching is a safe practice, and I guess this was her lesson. She learned that alignment according to your body is so important and knows when to rest and it's okay to rest. Keeping students safe during yoga practice is important, knowing how to modify a pose is key and knowing when a body is ready to do a certain pose can help save someone from injury.

My journey into yoga started one day during a golf lesson, the golf professional told me my spine was tight and so I should go to yoga, it was affecting my golf swing. What I did not know is that this advice would change my life forever. I followed his instructions and kept going to yoga, it was one of the hardest things I did but I kept coming back as I felt so amazing after class, and I fell in love with yoga. After about six months off work, I was keen to get back to work. I have always found it hard not working. I felt like I did not have a purpose. I was not sure what exactly I wanted to do so I decided to take a teacher training course in yoga in 2006, then maybe I could learn more about yoga. I loved the course, the people, the idea about yoga and just everything. Each weekend the course was on I was so excited and I would come home sore but happy. If only I knew then that this was going to be my life path, and that life was about to change. My body was tight; it was hard and still is. This was the start of a huge change for me on many levels, which I did not know at the time, which to be honest is common with most people.

By 2007, I had completed my first yoga teacher-training course. The course was a vinyasa flow course and I loved every minute of it, I felt we covered a broad spectrum of areas of teaching yoga, apart from actual practice teaching. At the end of the course, I had spent maybe less than 20 minutes teaching, so once I started to teach in the big wide world I realised how hard it actually was. Some of the ladies at the golf club asked me to teach them and I managed to build up a few classes. It was slow going but it always is if you are a new teacher. Especially if you are a teacher with a super tight body that can't do all the fancy poses. I made all the mistakes that all new teachers make but I was passionate and kind and wanted to learn and know more.

After a period of time teaching, I went to a hot yoga class, and I fell in love with it. It was much easier for me than ashtanga yoga as the heat helped my tight body and the poses did not seem as difficult. The feeling I experienced when I left the studio could not be put into words; I just felt amazing.

I decided I needed more training and I wanted to learn more about hot yoga. I found a course in Thailand, which suited my needs, and the idea of going to Thailand really appealed to me. So October 2008, I headed to Thailand and spent one-month training to become a hot yoga teacher. Having done a course before and some experience teaching, I felt I had a slight advantage, as I knew roughly how to teach but this course taught me so much more. It was one of the hardest things I did physically, emotionally and mentally but I loved it and it represents some of the best times of my life. The course was great but I did see flaws in the course, what did I know, I was super confident and I said one day I will run this course. I don't remember saying that but I have been reminded several times that apparently I did. I was growing confident, and my career was looking good.

During that trip, I spent some time in Bangkok and took some classes at a studio called, 'Absolute You', that's when I first met Luke. He was a cool guy from the USA he seemed to know a lot about yoga, and his classes seemed popular too, I tried to get a job at Absolute Yoga but it never worked, everyone ignored my emails, *Oh well it's not meant to be*, I figured. I went back to the UK and started to work hard at teaching hot yoga and I was very successful with it. A year later, I was back in Thailand for a friend's wedding and I got the chance to interview again for Absolute Yoga. I was put on schedule to teach a class and a senior teacher was due to attend my class and assess me. Long story short, the teacher forgot to come so I taught a class for no reason. I was asked to teach again two days later; they asked if I could take over Luke's hot flow class. Luke had been in Bangkok a few years or so and I have no idea what level to teach and I don't even know if anyone understands English. However, I wanted to work for 'Absolute You' so I did it. I taught hot flow and this time I had so many teachers in class as well as the company's owner; it was so nerve-racking. Somehow I made it through demonstrating everything and was fairly much out of breath most of the time from running around and talking so much. Lucky for me Luke said I did a good job.

Two months later, I found myself back in Thailand working full-time for the very company that I trained with on the TT course. I left the UK and embarked on a new life abroad. I settled right into this new life in Bangkok, and soon after I started teaching, I signed up for a Pilates Mat and Reformer training course. I had never liked pilates previously; I think because I never understood it, but this time it impacted me in a big way. I saw my body change through the practice and I learned so much.

In 2011, one of the team members of the hot teacher-training course, which I had taken previously, decided they were going to leave Thailand and so another team member was needed for the training course and I was asked to fill that role. I could not imagine, I was a student of the course and now I was going to become a trainer. I was so happy and excited but also nervous. I knew I had to prove myself. I, of course, made many mistakes and tried to be too good like we all do when we are new teachers.

My first course as a trainer was in 2011 and again, I loved every minute of it. By the time I came to the second course, I was more confident as I was given more duties. Each time I got better because in between the courses, I studied hard and attended more courses myself. After having completed three courses, the current course director decided to leave and I was appointed the course director of the training course. It was a huge task and of course, I made mistakes as we all do, it's the only way to grow. My first job was to edit manuals. I felt that they lacked some important information that teachers needed. I had taken a number of courses myself by this point and so my knowledge had expanded immensely. The first course I managed was TT11, even from day one there was drama and it was a sure test of many parts of my character and of course I made mistakes but each course got better and so did I.

I was a student in the hot teacher-training course in 2008 and by 2011, I was the course director and my final Hot TT training was in 2017. I had completed 14 hot yoga teacher-training courses with hundreds of students. In 2017, I moved from Bangkok to Barcelona to help set up a teacher training college. During the one year I spent in Spain, I helped manage a number of yoga training courses including, vinyasa, trapeze and hot yoga. All in all, I have helped manage or run about 30 training courses for people from all over the world. I have learned so much about myself, about teaching and running training courses.

Chapter 2
Role of the Teacher

Every time I run a teacher training this question will always come up: is it a yoga teacher or a yoga instructor. My thoughts are that it doesn't really matter, but let's examine each option anyway.

A 'teacher' is a person who helps students to acquire knowledge. A teacher often works in a classroom. An instructor is a person who teaches something. So it's the same, at least not exactly. The two words are interchangeable, but there's a small difference. When you teach, you impart knowledge, whereas when you instruct, you impart skills. Therefore, a teacher is one who teaches you about a subject and helps you to understand the subject, and an instructor is one who instructs you on how to accomplish a task.

So which is correct, both I would say, we do guide people through poses and help them do the pose to the best of their abilities. But sometimes, we do teach them something i.e., maybe something about the knee joint they did not know. So honestly titles and names don't matter, it's what your intention is that matters and don't get bogged down with small details such as names.

The role of the teacher

In essence, the role of the teacher is to teach a yoga class. Moving students through a number of poses. In order to do this, we need to have a good understanding of the purpose of the yoga pose and how students can achieve it. Moving from a start position into a yoga pose involves moving a number of joints and if we don't know enough about what is the purpose of a pose or how to modify it then we can do more damage than good. It's important to know that you can't learn all this information in your first course, or your first year of teaching, it takes a lifetime. Simply embarking on a journey of becoming a yoga teacher in the west takes one 200 course and then some teaching time. Of course, this is all you need to do and you can continue to teach for the rest of your life.

But if you want to become a great teacher and keep up to date with new ideas, you need to keep studying. Information I was given years back does not make sense in the world we live in today. Understanding the cues that were used many years ago might not work for today's world and current students.

The first training course I took was great, but in reality, we can't take it all in the first time around, it's all too much new information at once, hence I decided to write a book. The aim of this book is for teachers who have been teaching anything from six months to 20 years and who would like to refine their teaching. I have some great simple tips that can change the way you teach in a short period of time. I teach much of this during my training courses but the reality is, there is so much information to take in that not everything can be consumed during the one-month training. I believe as people who work with people's bodies we should continue to learn and keep up to date. Which requires us teachers to continue to study and attend training courses.

Let's get back to the basic role of the teacher is to guide a group of people through their yoga practice safely. Sounds simple enough but we often get caught up with other ideas like how to make people laugh or how to make the class fancy, or how I make students like me and my class.

You'll be surprised that the class does not need to be as fancy as you think. You don't need to use fancy words and you don't need to wear fancy yoga clothes. These are all things we get caught up in thinking we need to do these things. Does it help make you a better teacher if you have the latest season in yoga pants? It might make you feel confident if you look good in the pants but even if you are bad at teaching, fancy pants won't save you.

I decided after my first TT course, I would use the Sanskrit names or poses so I sounded like I knew what I was saying. Forinstance, Trianga Mukhaikapada Paschimottanasana sounds way fancier than the half-hero pose. The reality is after I announce the fancy Sanskrit name, I always follow it with the English name because no one knows what it is and it takes so long to say the name, so often best just to say the English name. I'm not saying don't use Sanskrit names; I do use some names it's understanding why we say them. I said it because I wanted to sound fancy like a yoga teacher that's maybe not the best reason. Especially as new teachers, we want to be the best and we often feel that by using fancy words it will make us sound more experienced or sound like a better teacher. When in reality, all we need to know is how to teach a good class using words that make sense to our audience.

Then, of course, you can go down the route of talking about prana, life force, and chakras. I am not saying any of this is wrong I am saying don't say it for the sake of trying to sound like a yoga teacher. You also need to understand your audience and whether it is appropriate to them. I found when I talked to some of the guys at the golf club, I would talk about yoga more in terms of a stretch class rather than a mind-body connection as I knew they did not understand it and had no interest. They simply wanted to know how it would improve their golf game.

Once you get more confident in teaching these are great things to include in your classes, but make sure you understand what you are talking about. Sometimes this is a great way to find a focus for your class. I.e., in today's class, we will focus on opening the throat chakra including poses that fit the theme and maybe talk about reasons why the throat chakra might be blocked, explain where it is and why it's good to activate the throat chakra. It's easy to throw a bunch of these spiritual words and phrases around to sound more like a yoga teacher but times have changed and teaching yoga has changed. Previously it was always thought that yogis were hippies, incense-burning people who wear baggy colourful pants and carry crystals and beads. Today yoga has a different image and the image of yoga teachers is very different. Doctors often refer people to go to yoga to help heal bad backs and to deal with stress. As yoga continues to grow, the image changes and we as teachers need to adjust to the current climate.

Another trap we fall into is spouting anatomy as this will also make us look like we are good teachers. This is a very important area to fully understand and know what you are talking about. Of course, saying that feel your hamstrings stretching is good and most people will understand it. But to start talking about engaging your serratus anterior to stabilise your shoulders probably won't work because:

1. What is that and where is it?
2. How do I engage it?
3. Why do I need to stabilise my shoulders?
4. How do I know if it's engaged or not?

Understand your audience. If you are teaching a group of yoga teachers, maybe this works, but new students often don't even know which is their right or left leg. I think it's good to educate students on the anatomy of the body and to get them to understand the purpose of each pose and what muscles are working and how, but you don't want your yoga class to sound like an anatomy class for doctors. You also need to make sure if you do say something about anatomy that you get it right i.e., know the action of the muscle and what is happening is it stretching or strengthening. Students sometimes will come and speak after class and might say, "When I am in this pose I feel this." It's important you have an understanding of anatomy and what is happening in the pose so you know if students feel the right thing. I personally feel that most yoga teachers are not educated enough in anatomy, we are working with people's bodies and it's important we should know what is going on. We should know what the position of the hip in warrior 2 is and also understand what muscles create the movement. I know many teachers who have been teaching for 15 years or more and don't know what muscles are used to create external rotation of the hip. If you are working with people's bodies, it is important to know how they work.

As a yoga teacher, you have an audience and as humans, we always want to please our audience as we want them to like us. So, do we need to be funny and tell jokes in class, or maybe we should be strict and serious? Finding out who you are as a teacher takes time and we are often not our true selves for the first year as we are so focused on trying to get through the class, saying the words and remembering the sequence. Adding in humour might not be something that you will include until you feel very comfortable teaching. You also don't need to be funny to be liked by some people like more serious teachers.

Most people fall into the strict and serious bracket to start with. Especially when we first teach it's very difficult and we want to make every class the best so we feel we need to control the class, we must control the class and you must do what I say. This happens generally because we are serious about wanting to make this newfound career work and much like any job we take it seriously and then become serious. Which I am not saying is wrong, I believe anyone who takes his or her job seriously is on the right path.

Of course, everyone is different in what they prefer, and some do like a serious teacher who is strict. I personally think we are not in the military so why do we need to be so strict. Of course, there is always the argument about building focus and concentration, which I do believe is important, but for me, there is so much more involved. I can remember going to a hot yoga class once and the rules were strict about drinking water when you can sit down and have to have the towel on the mat. I did not want my towel on my mat; I did not sweat so much and I felt the mat gave me more grip but the teacher insisted. That was the rules and okay fair enough but not every rule works for everybody and this is just a yoga class after all. The teacher was ex-military so it made sense that he taught that way. I also don't agree of having a free-for-all, everyone do what they want, I just think there is a way to deliver the information and also understand when you can relax a bit and not be so strict.

Your favourite teacher versus your least favourite

I want you to think about your favourite teacher and answer some questions. What is it you like about this teacher's class?

- Is the teacher friendly?
- Does the teacher adjust students?
- Do they offer options/modifications?
- Is it okay to rest in class?
- Do they know your name?
- Did they start and finish on time?
- Are they consistent?
- Did they play music?
- How was the sequence?
- Did they talk to you before or after class?

Think about your answers to the questions above and write them on a piece of paper, think about which is most important. Now place them in the order of importance to you.

This will help give you an idea of what you should focus on when you teach.

Now consider a class you went to that you did not like and think about these questions:

- Did they talk too much or too little?
- Did they adjust students?
- How was their sequence?
- Do they offer options/modifications?
- Was it too easy or too hard?
- Did the teacher practice the class?
- How was their voice tone?
- Did they set up the pose correctly?
- What is it specifically that you didn't like?
- Was the teacher friendly?

Now place them in the order of importance to you. This will help give you an idea of what you should not focus on when you teach. You can learn so much not only from classes you that you like but also from those classes you don't enjoy. When I was training, I took classes with lots of different teachers and noted things I liked and did not like and added that to my teaching. The reality is if we like a teacher or we enjoy their class, we will often forgive simple mistakes, as the rest of the experience is so good. However, if we don't like a teacher, we'll notice every tiny thing they do, possibly even the way they pronounce a word. Unless you have good control of your mind, it's hard to find things that you like, and we get focused on the small things. We are often drawn to a teacher because they're similar to us, i.e., strong and commanding, or calm and relaxed. I've found through my training courses that most people tend to teach the style of class they prefer to practice. I like a strong class and if the teacher is too calm and does not push me, I find it hard to push myself. I like a tough workout and so I tend to teach in a similar way. However, I don't take myself too seriously and I always like to include some humour and lightness in the class.

So how do you know what sort of teacher you are, there are no rules, you don't have to fit into some bracket you just need to be true to yourself. When I train teachers, I say to them don't aim to teach like me I have been doing this for 17 years. I tell them they might not be the best at what they do but if you are nice; you deliver a good class and people enjoy themselves then you are on the way to teaching a good class.

If your students were to describe your class, what would you like to hear them say?

If I was to answer that question, I would like people to say the class was a strong well-planned class, the teacher was kind/caring and the class was fun. Notice I did not say what a great body the teacher has or what a great practice the teacher has. That's because those things are not important to me. I want students to have left my class feeling different in their bodies or mind and having had some fun. A fun class will always go faster than a dull, boring class. When students look at the clock, either the class is too hard or too dull.

So we looked at things about our favourite teacher and some things that we did not like about a certain teacher's class. Let's examine the teacher you liked:

- Did they have an amazing body?
- Were they super flexible or strong?

- Were they super charismatic?
- Were they wearing the latest brand of yoga pants?

The reality is the most successful teachers are not different to you they just have more experience. Your practice will never be perfect, but you keep working on it to keep improving. You don't need to be perfect, you just need to continue to grow so your students get inspired to grow with you. Not everyone can look like a model and do every pose to perfection but we can grow to learn to be great yoga teachers.

What you should focus on is:

- Your practice.
- Learning and continued study.
- Selfless intent to help others.
- Connection and community with your students.

In reality, you need to know a little bit more than your students; you need to have a little bit more experience and a bit more energy and excitement. Think about your teaching, list five things you think you are good at and then list five things you think you could improve on. Then make it your goal to focus your mind on the things you are good at but your intention to improve the things you are not so good at. Don't focus on the negatives focus on the positives. Things that you could improve on are not negatives they are simply areas where you need to refine your skills.

How to teach a yoga class

In essence, the basic role is to teach a class and in order to do that, a teacher should know a number of basic things. Below are some basic points that you need to consider when teaching a class as a newish teacher, however after a period of time teaching you need to consider other aspects of planning a class like the order of pose in terms of standing series, seated, prone, etc.

- What is the pose name?
- What is the setup/alignment for a pose?
- What is the purpose?
- What parts of the body should be mobilised first?
- How to design a basic class?

There are of course many other factors to consider which I will expand on further later on in the book such as dialogue, adjustments etc.

In terms of timing, make sure you start and finish on time. You might not think this is important but it actually is. Does it matter if you go over five minutes to give students a longer savasana? It can.

One of the hidden aspects of yoga, which we learn through the practice of yoga, is discipline. We keep coming back to the practice in order to achieve a stronger body, a more flexible body or to get closer to achieving a certain pose. So if we expect students to be disciplined in taking their practice seriously by not talking in class or dedicating time to practice etc. We should also ensure we are disciplined in our approach to teaching, which means starting on time. Traffic is never an excuse to be late, I live in Bangkok the traffic is bad and always has been. Some days are worse than others. So always make sure you have time to arrive at the studio. I will always arrive a minimum of 30 minutes before that way if I encounter a problem, chances are I will arrive on time as opposed to being late. Of course, there are always unforeseen circumstances like road closures etc. However, in day-to-day as a teacher, we should be at the studio before class starts thus enabling us the chance to talk to students before class starts, check the microphone is working and prepare our minds for the class ahead.

Finishing on time is often even more important for many reasons. If there is a class after yours, you need to finish on time in order to give the next teacher time to set up for their class or prepare for setting up the room. Students might be on a limited parking time, or they have limited time i.e., for a lunchtime class, they might need to get back to work. If you find halfway through class you might go over time, then you need to speed things up or cut poses out.

Is it okay to finish early? In simple terms no it's not okay. Of course, 2–3 minutes early is okay but 5–10 minutes is not acceptable. Lots of classes these days are 60 minutes only so if you cut that short to 50 minutes students have lost about 16% of the class.

There is no reason to finish early if you find your class has finished early you can make the final relaxation longer or maybe add in some breathing exercises. No two classes are the same, you can prepare a 60 minutes sequence and with two different groups, it can be too long or too short. When you have a group of strong students who know what they are doing, things tend to move faster. However, a group with some beginners might take longer as they might need more help or time spent with adjustments etc. Always have a backup plan, i.e., extra poses up your sleeve that makes sense to add in at the end if you finish earlier than expected.

As movement specialists, our role as teachers is to ensure everyone is safe. This might mean that at some points in class, the more experienced students may need to hold a pose or wait whilst you fix a new student. Of course, it's not right to keep people waiting for one student only unless they are compromised i.e., they could hurt themselves. Not going deep into a pose does not count but if someone falls during an arm balance you need to ensure they are okay before you move on. That often just involves eye contact and asking them, "Are you okay?" If they are, you continue if not then maybe have everyone take the Child's pose or give them a water break whilst you check on the student. I don't believe you should keep the group waiting for one student but if something has happened and they need your attention then, of course, you should, i.e., someone faints in class or has fallen and hurt themselves. If their feet are not perfectly parallel and they don't seem to understand the cue, don't have everyone else wait whilst you fix the issues, especially small ones.

After teacher training

Of course, the reality is teaching is very different to practising and some don't realise that until they take a teacher training course. It becomes a dream of many to live in this new, fabulous world. Living in the yoga world with like-minded people doing yoga daily wearing mala beads and chanting mantras to get enlightened. Sounds fun, but it's not exactly like this.

The reality is it's a job like other jobs but we are changing lives and seeing people improve their postures their health and much more. Yoga over other forms of fitness does tend to attract a different group of people. Many times I have had students who know better, who start to do something different to everyone else. They are 'an advanced student', honestly, I don't even know what that means because despite practising for many years, I am not an advanced student. Does it mean you can do advanced poses? The reality is there are many reasons why someone can't do a pose. Anyone who says they are advanced, generally are not. A guru in India might be considered an advanced student but if you were to ask them, they would probably say they are just a student and teacher.

Teacher training is a new experience for most and brings much joy in many ways. It's a test on all levels, physical, emotional and mental. Being away from home is hard for some people, the constant practice, the long days and the lack of sleep. The constant study and teaching, the sitting all day, it can be exhausting. However, it can be magical, inspiring and life-changing. The soreness in the hips or back will disappear but the magic of the journey will stay with you forever.

So once teacher training is finished, real life begins and reality hits. Most are keen to teach to start to earn money back and maybe recover the costs of the training course. Or even simply to just start teaching. As a new teacher, it's hard to get classes as everyone knows you're new. So the best way is to offer to cover classes but in reality, no one wants a new teacher. I know, I went through this whole journey myself.

You need to teach to get better but no one wants you. Much like most things in life, this will change over time. After training is done, the key thing is to earn some money to recover the costs of the teacher-training course. We get so involved in the teaching part that we often forget about our own practice. We sacrifice our practice in order to teach; I know I did it too.

The study, of course, is important but practice teaches you so much. Some of the best lessons can come from your own practice. Learning what works for you and how you modify it to achieve a pose. Learning why something is difficult or easy for you can help you understand the journey of your students. A book can teach you what muscles are contracted or stretched but practise can tell you how it feels in the body. It helps you understand if the feeling is a good stretch feeling or if it's more towards a pain that might not be good. I always say on teacher training the day before graduation that you will miss the double class per day. At a time when everyone is sore and a bit sick of practise, there is an element of relief from a break from doing double classes every day. However, once normal life returns just getting to one class per day is a challenge and that's when people realise what I meant. Keeping up your own practice along with teaching is hard, demonstrating the odd pose when you teach does not count as practice.

Part of being a good yoga teacher is keeping up with your own personal practice. The thing that brings lots of people to teaching yoga is initially the love of yoga and how it makes them feel. Sometimes a class is easy and sometimes the easiest of classes can be a struggle. The sense of achievement when you can finally do a pose that was difficult or just the feeling of pure joy after class. It becomes part of your life and life somehow changes. I could never describe the feeling after a hot yoga class, I just felt great but I could not put my finger on what it was exactly but that feeling was addictive.

Practise is about having full attention to your body on your mat and going through whatever class or sequence it is that day. Does it need to be daily or three times a week? My answer is always simple more is always better. Three times a week is better than two and five is better than three. Repetition is key for anything in life. If you want to learn a language, keep repeating and studying will get you there faster. If you want to achieve the splits, you need to work on it as much as you can. If you can only give 10 mins per day, then make that happen, five sun salutations are always better than nothing and you will be surprised once you start, you might even continue a little further. As teachers, we should practise what we preach otherwise we are not setting a good example for our students. I also believe there is always time, it might mean getting up 30 minutes earlier but it's about choices. Don't get me wrong I do not get up at 4 am to practice but I know people that do. I myself have also had times in my life where I have lost my practice, so what I do now is I make the goal smaller, so it's achievable. Rather than saying I will do full primary series five times a week, I commit to a standing series 3–5 times a week, in reality, it always goes further or maybe I go take a hot yoga class. The fact that I know I only need to commit x amount of time and I know it will happen.

Practice is different for everyone. It can be taking a class or self-practice. It does not need to look like a specific set thing i.e., it does not need to be the full primary series every time. It needs to be some version of what you need.

Understanding how your body feels different every day and it needs different things can help you connect with students' feelings. So, think about your own practice what does it look like? Are you happy with the amount you do and the effort you put in? Do your students practice more than you? Most of your students have full-time jobs they work 40 hours a week. For yoga teachers, we might teach 15 classes per week. If we assume all classes are 90 minutes, that's 22.5 hours plus some class prep time which is less than most working people. These days' lots of studios have lots of 60-minute classes so in actuality it could be less. It might be my perspective but we can always make time for things we really want. It's just down to how much we really want it. You can choose to sleep longer or you can choose to wake up earlier and practice if only for 20 minutes.

You can't give from an empty cup so although teaching 25 classes per week might bring lots of cash, but will the 25th class be as good as the first? It should be because you should give 100% in every class but the reality is we get tired. Teaching yoga takes a lot of physical and emotional energy. I am very guilty of teaching too much it's part of my nature to work hard. I do however make time for me. It might not be specifically 90 mins of yoga every day but it's some sort of movement that helps my emotional, mental and physical sanity. As I have got older I realise less work and more time for other things is so important.

This lockdown time was a great time for me to step back and look at things. Having had lots of time off work due to taking care of my sick mum there was part of me that felt I needed to make up for what I missed which meant working hard in my mind but actually, COVID taught me the opposite.

Take time for me more and it's okay to not be the say yes to everything person. It's been a passion of mine to write a book in order to help people achieve their dreams so taking time to write this is every bit as important as teaching students.

I often refer to yoga as sneaky as once yoga is part of your life other life choices seem to improve. We decide not to go out and party on Friday night because we want to go to yoga on Saturday morning. After the morning class is done, fried chicken and a bottle of wine does not seem as appealing a choice for lunch as maybe a Greek salad and watermelon shake. Okay, I know what you're thinking there is nothing wrong with fried chicken and a bottle of wine, and personally, there is nothing I like more than a cold glass of white wine. But when you start to ask for an early dinner or you don't fancy going to the disco because you want to be able to go to class, that's when it's got you. Yoga sneaks in the back door and helps improve life in so many ways. This whole feeling of awesomeness often steers people towards teacher training.

Chapter 3
Understanding Poses

Understanding yoga poses

In order to know how to set up, teach and modify a pose you need to know what is going on in a pose. What is the purpose of the pose, i.e., is it to stretch the hamstrings or open the hips. For instance, butterfly pose (baddha konasana) the purpose of the pose is to open the hips in external rotation whilst stretching the inner thighs. So as teachers we should know why this movement is important plus also why for some students it's easy and for some it's difficult. If you understand a pose, then you can also offer modifications easier because you know what the essence is, in this case, it's opening the hips in external rotation, so is there another way the same goal can be achieved if someone finds this pose too difficult.

It's very important we know what is happening anatomically in a pose, if we know this we can understand better how to adjust students and also understand why it's easy for some and not others. For instance, why is it that someone who cycles might find a butterfly pose difficult, whereas ballet dancers tend to find it much easier. Having this sort of information is extremely useful for a teacher. How much detail do you need to know? It's like personal practice the more you know the better. Understanding the basic function of the muscle or the purpose of a pose is key. You don't need to know small details such as inserts and origins of muscles but will it help if you do? Of course, it will. The more you know the better equipped you are to deal with people's bodies. Anatomy for me is an important subject as I believe many teachers don't know enough. It's not enough to simply know that your hamstrings are stretching in a seated forward fold, but what do you do if someone comes to you with an injury to one of the hamstrings. If a student brings a report from a doctor that says I have a spinal issue and the L5 disk is herniated anteriorly? What can they do or not do? Potentially the wrong decision can make it a lot worse, hence we need to have a good idea about the body. If you don't know it all now, it's not a problem you have time, study one pose at a time and you will be amazed at what you can learn in one month.

Why are some poses difficult or easy for some people?

We need to understand that everybody has a different body structure and even if two people look the same their poses might look different. Understanding a person's history of the movement and possible career choices can affect how someone's body moves. For instance, a hairdresser or chef tends to be rounded forward for their job, the chances are spinal flexion will be easier for them whereas extension might be more challenging. They may also experience lower back pain from standing all day in a flexed position. So for this type of student core strength, posterior chain strength and spinal mobility is key.

People who sit at a desk all day may also experience lower back pain, tight hamstrings and tight hip flexors due to being in a seated position all day.

Other considerations are tight ligaments or fascia, limb length and bone compression all of which can affect mobility. It's much easier to bind in a pose when you have long arms.

So how do you know what the issue is? I.e., are the hamstring tight or is it tightness in the lower back or weak hip flexors. Understanding this takes further investigation and observation of students' movements through various poses. This also takes the experience of seeing different bodies over time. Let's examine a seated forward fold and the possibilities of what could be wrong. When someone rounds their back in a seated forward fold, where is the tightness? Is it the hamstrings, lower back or weak hip flexors? The best way to find out is to take one of the possibilities out of the equation and see what changes.

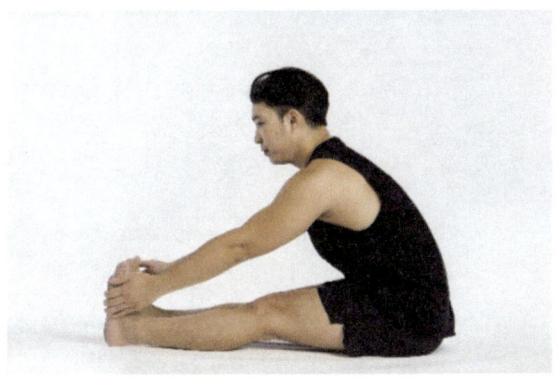

Paschimottanasana

Option 1 – Ask them to bend their knees and see if they can fold forward more or check if their back position improves, it could be tight hamstrings. You can also see them in other poses where the hamstrings are being stretched and see how they are with it, do they struggle? Or is it easy?

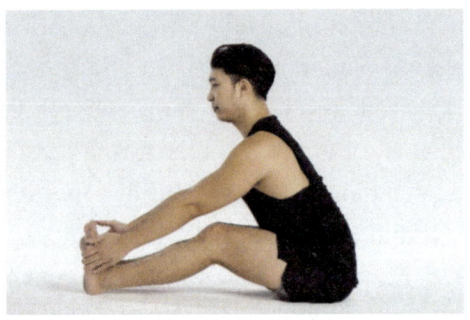

Pashimottanasana

Option 2 – Sit them on a block and see if they have less tension in their hip flexors. The block changes the angle of the hip so it's not so flexed, which can release hip flexor gripping. You can also offer a strap to see if they can lengthen their back.

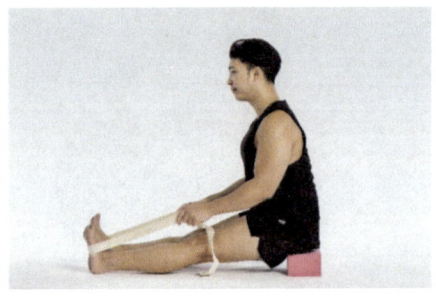

Pashimottanasana

If you take the back out of the equation i.e., do a different hamstring stretch, you can easily see if it's a tight back. (Big toe poses supine.)

Also, check that they are moving from the hip and not the lower back, you can also do the same thing standing hinge forward at the hips and see if you can touch the floor.

These are general ideas for things to look at, the picture is much bigger though because it could be a bone compression issue and much more. The first thing is to ask the student what do they feel, they might simply say, "My hamstrings are so tight," then you possibly have your answer so know how to modify it so they feel the stretch but are more comfortable with the level.

Knowing modifications

As a teacher, you need to know how to modify a pose, generally, modifications tend to be for someone who has an injury or for someone who simply can't achieve the pose. So this might mean to digress i.e., make it easier or more accessible, find a pose that can achieve the same result but it's easier to achieve. A simple pose like a butterfly can be super difficult for someone with tight hips, giving the student a block to sit on can make it feel much more comfortable.

Modifications can also mean progression, i.e., make it more challenging. Someone simply might not feel anything in the pose and although this is okay, if you do know a way to make the student feel something then it's good to offer that option. As an example in paschimottanasana if they can reach their feet and don't feel their hamstrings, a good option might be to give them a block and place it in front of their feet and have them pull back on the block to intensify the stretch. You can't of course run around the room modifying for every student. But once you teach someone a modification, you can explain to them they can do it each time they are in your class. I say your class because it's something you have offered them other teachers might not be happy about it hence, I always say to students when in my class you can do this.

Most of the time, I have found modifications are for people who have injuries or limitations. They may have had surgery or had an accident. For example, someone with a plate in their knee might not be able to bend the knee fully so a pigeon pose might be available to them. So you need to know how to modify otherwise, a student is left sitting there watching others. In this case, maybe a figure of four pose or supine pigeon supine might be better as the knee does not need to be flexed to the same degree.

Downward Dog

So let's examine Downward Dog, a pose often taught in yoga and sometimes as a transition pose.

Firstly, when we talk about what is happening in a pose i.e., hips flexed etc. we need to have a start position. This position is called the anatomical position. So, this would be the start position and then we move from there.

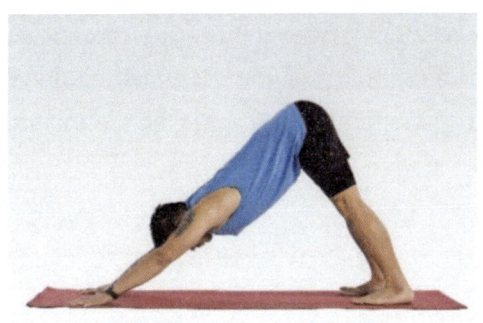

Downward Dog

What is anatomical position, the body is standing upright, with the feet at shoulder width and parallel, toes forward. The upper limbs are held out to each side, and the palms of the hands face forward. This is the start position and in yoga, we often refer to this as the mountain pose. From here, we move into a pose. So what do we need to know about a pose?

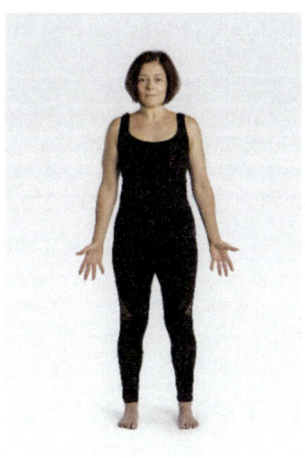

Anatomical Position

So what is happening in Downward Dog? Firstly, let's look at the position of the joints. Movement occurs at the joints, if we know what position the joints should be in we can easily tell if something is wrong when someone has their joints in the wrong set-up.

Joint Position

Hips – Flexed
Knees – Extended
Shoulders – Flexed and externally rotated
Elbows – Extended
Forearms – Pronated
Wrist – Dorsi flexed
Cervical spine – Flexed
Lumbar – Extends

The joint mobility is determined by muscles, ligaments, fascia and bone structure. The thing that should be looked at first is the muscles, as muscles can help move the bones and if it's just muscle tightness, then stretching can help change things.

When we talk about muscles, there are four types of ways in which muscles work, we will mainly focus on the first two.

- Agonist – The prime mover responsible for movement.
- Antagonist – The muscle that works in opposition of the agonist.
- Stabiliser – The muscle that stabilises the joint.

- Synergist – They assist the agonist but are not the prime mover.

For instance, in a biceps curl, the prime mover is the biceps and the antagonist is the triceps. What that means is when one muscle contracts i.e., the biceps the triceps will relax. So if you want to stretch or lengthen your hamstrings more, then you would contract your quadriceps.

It's important we need to know the opposing muscle group as quite often if one group is strong or tight the opposing muscle group could be weaker. In my case, my hip flexors are strong and my hip extensors are weaker. So for me to flex my hips is pretty straightforward whereas for someone else it might be more challenging. Although flexing my hips is straightforward, I am still limited by the tightness in my hip extensors so no matter how strong one muscle group is, if another is tight the range of motion can still be limited. A tight muscle does not mean it's strong. It can be tight and weak but also tight and strong.

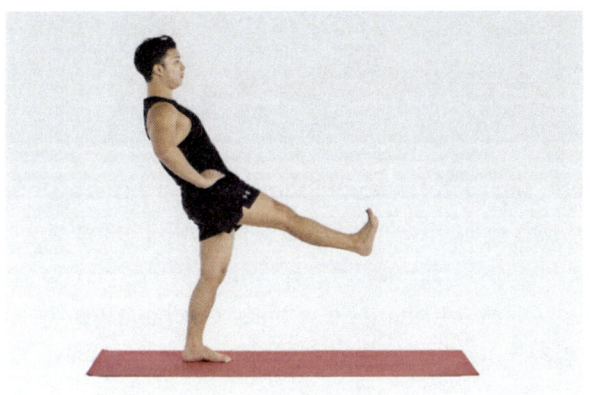

Single Leg Lift

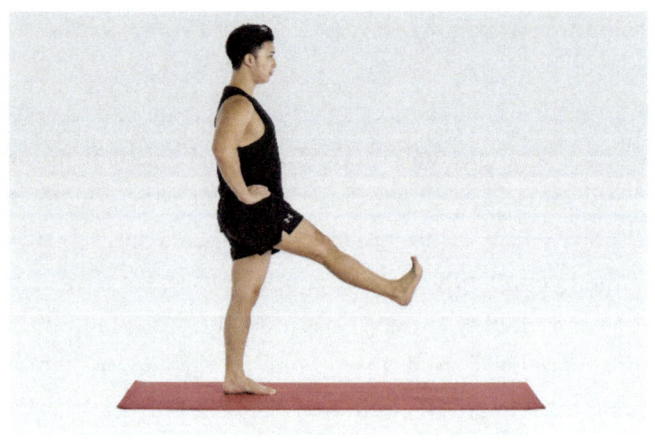

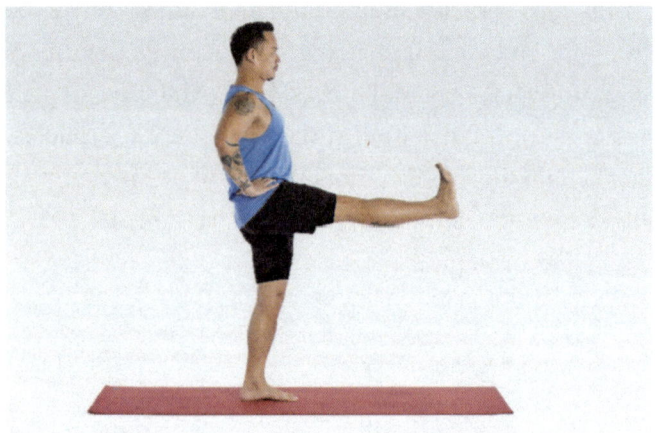

See in the pictures above the height of the leg differs, in fact, in both cases they are strong but one person has tighter hip extensors which make it harder to lift the leg and you can see when Flynn lift the leg the body compensates by leaning back. When he leans back, it does not improve his hip flexibility at all; he is doing it to compensate for the lack of mobility. So it's better to keep the leg lower and work on mobility in other poses too.

Downward Dog

Hips

Prime mover for flexing the hips – iliacus, psoas and rectus femoris. The hip flexors **Opposing muscle group** – hamstrings (semimembranosus, semitendinosus, biceps femoris) and gluteus maximus. The hip extensors.

Knees

The prime mover that extends the knee are the quadriceps (rectus femoris, vastus lateralis, vastus medius, and vastus intermedius).

The opposing muscle group is the hamstrings (semimembranosus, semitendinosus, biceps femoris) so if they are tight it might not be possible to fully extend the knee. So the legs might not be fully straight. If the hamstring group is tight, it can also lead to rounding in the lower back.

When we talk about straight, what are we talking about? We are talking about the alignment of the bones so for a leg to be straight, the ankle, knee and hip bones will be in one perfect line. These bony landmarks help us to see if there is a deviation from the neutral position. So if the knee joint is neutral the greater trochanter (hip bone), lateral epicondyle (knee bone) and lateral malleolus (ankle bone) would be in one straight line.

Muscles can affect the position of the bones so if the hamstrings are tight this could affect the position of the bones so the lateral epicondyle might be forward and not in line with the greater trochanter and lateral malleolus. Therefore, the knees would be flexed and the leg would not be perfectly straight. This can be common with runners who tend to have tight hamstrings. More common in yoga students is the opposite i.e., the knee bone is behind the hip and ankle bone so the knee is hyperextended. Which means the hamstrings need more strength. Most people experience either option without any issues or pain but the thing we want to work towards is using muscles to move and stabilise the joints and not relying on joint mobility.

Shoulders – Flexion

Prime mover – Anterior deltoid and pectoralis major.

The opposing muscle group latissimus dorsi and posterior deltoid. (Shoulder extensors)

If they are tight, it will be challenging to flex the shoulder. What tends to happen in this case is students will compensate for tight shoulders by extending the spine and pushing the ribcage forward, which actually means the shoulder does not open more it just means the abs are not engaged and the spine goes into extension. Which in itself defeats the object of opening the shoulders.

Shoulders – External rotation

Prime Mover – Infraspinatus and teres minor
The opposing muscle group – is the subscapularis which internally rotates the shoulder so if this is tight external rotation will be challenging. Also, if the humerus is internally rotated, it will make external rotation even more challenging.

Elbows – Extended

Prime Mover – Triceps brachii muscle extends the elbow
The opposing muscle group – is the elbow flexors biceps brachii, brachioradialis and brachialis. So if the elbow flexors, i.e., Biceps are tight and short then students might not be able to fully extend the elbow. You might see this with people who are very muscular, they are not able to fully extend the elbow.

Forearms – Pronation

In order to get the hands flat on the mat including the thumbs, you need to be able to pronate the forearm.

Prime Mover – Pronator teres and pronater quadratus.

The opposing muscle group – Biceps brachii and supinator are the supinators.

The other thing to consider is when you pronate the forearm the radius bone will cross over the ulna, once they hit each other there is nowhere to go, we call this bone compression and no matter how hard you try you cannot change this situation. Stretching of muscles will not help but understanding this might explain why it's hard for some people to press their thumbs down.

Wrist – Dorsi flexed

Prime Mover – that extends the wrist are extensor carpi radialis, longus and brevis, along with the extensor carpi ulnaris.

The opposing muscle group – are the flexors are flexor carpi, radialis, palmaris longus, flexor carpi ulnaris, and pronator teres. There can of course also be bone restriction which will limit the mobility in the joint.

Cervical spine – Flexed

Prime Mover – That flex the cervical spine are longus capitis, rectus capitis anterior and rectus capitis lateralis.

The opposing muscle group – The extensors are levator scapulae, upper trapezius, splenius capitis and cervis and semispinalis capitis and cervis.

These days we tend to have a lot of head forward posture from looking at digital devices and this will lengthen the flexors muscle. This constant head forward can put a lot of strain on the shoulders and back too.

Lumbar spine – Extends

Prime Mover – that extends the spine is the erector spinae, which includes iliocostalis, longissimus, and spinalis.

If the hip flexors are also tight, this may also pull the pelvis forward into an anterior tilt, thus also increasing the extension in the lumbar region.

The opposing muscle group – is the obliques and rectus abdominus.

Let's look at two bodies that look the same but their downward dogs are different. As you can see from the picture where they are standing, their body types are similar. But the downward dogs are slightly different due to muscle tightness

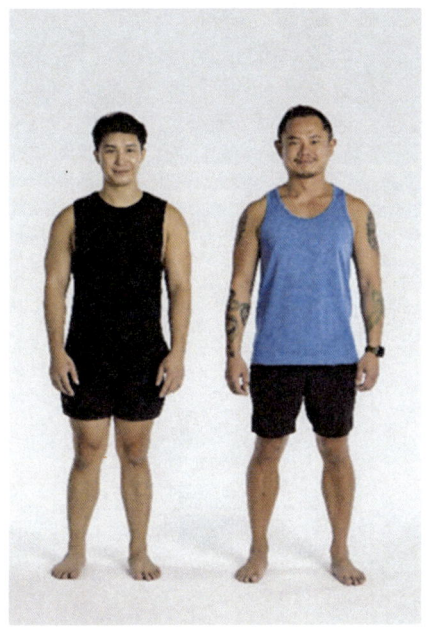

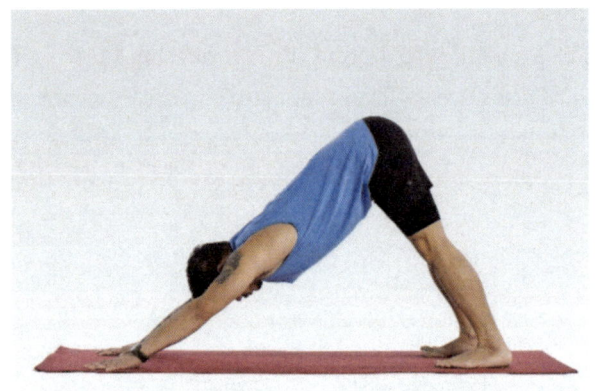

Downward Dog

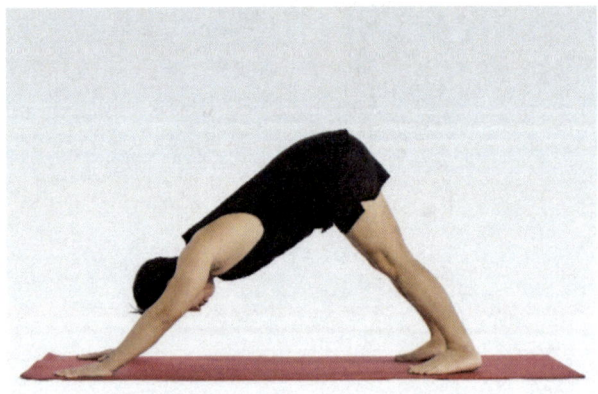

Downard Dog

So now we know what muscles are performing the action in order to achieve the pose, we know what needs to be lengthened and what needs to be strong. However, bones affect how a pose looks and we have to consider what tightness and what strength means. You can be tight i.e., have tight hamstrings but that does not mean that they are strong. Muscles can be tight and weak but also at the same time long and strong. So in order to achieve downward dog, one thing you do need is shoulder mobility but you also need arm strength in order to hold the pose.

So what are the benefits of a Downward Dog?

The shoulders, hips and back side of the body get stretched and opened specifically the hamstrings calves and shoulders. The arms and legs get strengthened there is also the added benefit of being slightly inverted so the heart is above the head so it does not need to work as hard to get blood flow to the brain.

How do you know if it is muscle tightness or something else?

This can take years of knowledge and practice and understanding of different bodies. A simple method would be to ask what restricts you if it's muscle they might say my hamstrings feel so tight, if it's a bone restriction the student might say I don't know I just can't go further. I have a bone restriction issue at my ankle so I can't get my heals down in downward dog, Once I change the angle of the ankle joint, I can get my heels down but then my downward dog is too short and I have too much pressure on my upper body.

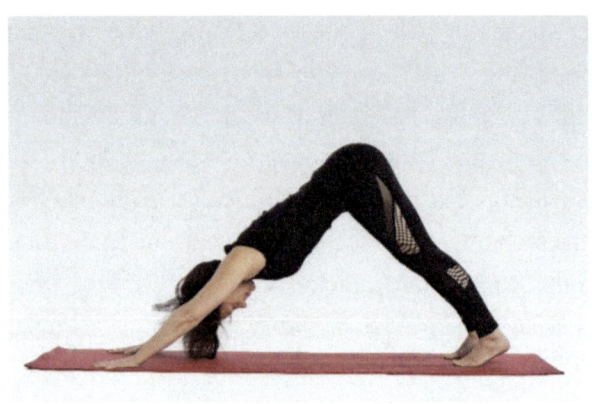

Downward Dog

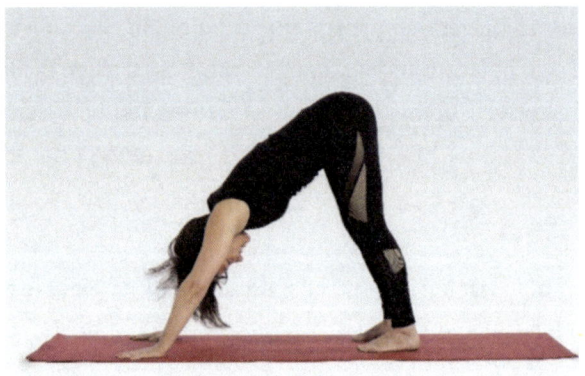

Downward Dog

It's very easy to work out the restriction when looking at other poses when you need ankle mobility. See awkward pose part 1 and part 2. You can see in part 2 that once I change the angle of the ankle joint, I have much more mobility. See picture 3 and you can see once I have heel support, which changes the angle of the ankle joint I can sit lower.

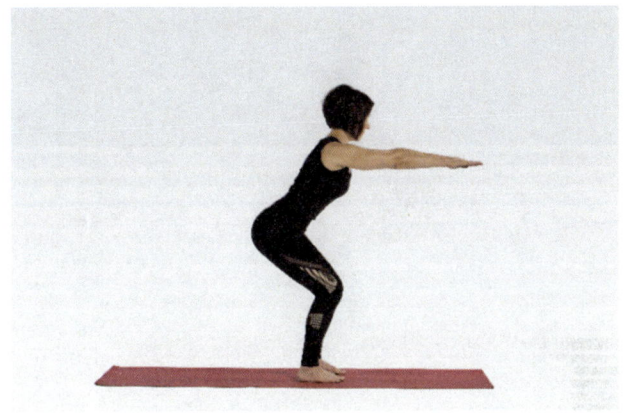

Awkward

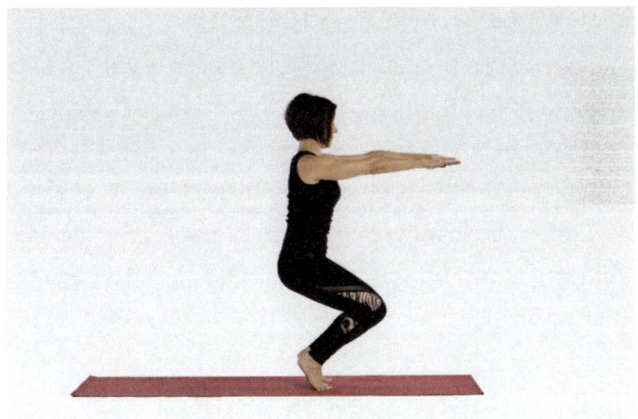

Awkward

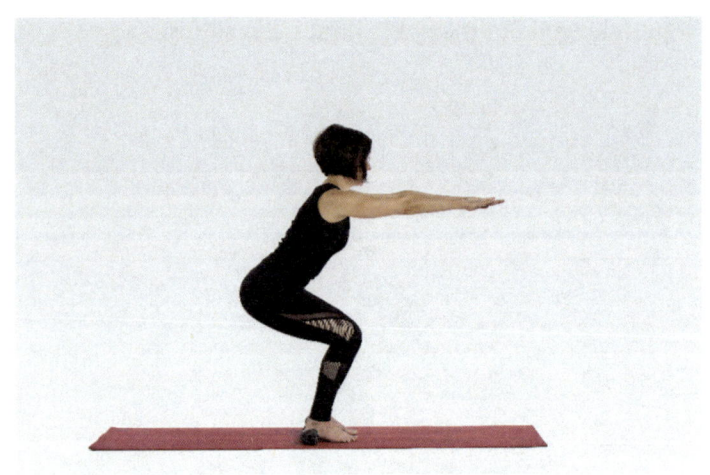

Awkward

How to modify Downward Dog

If someone has tight hamstrings, you can ask them to bend the knees to take pressure off the lower back. If their wrists are weak may be lower to the forearms. Place blocks or a yoga mat under their heels to help support the legs. You also add blocks under the hands to release pressure on the wrists. Sometimes a strap around the shoulder to help engage the shoulder stabilisers.

Mobility, stability and flexibility

As yoga teachers, we need to understand what needs to be mobile in order to achieve a pose and what needs to be stabilising. Mobility is more to do with muscle control and the joint and what range of motion you have, i.e., using muscles to control entry and exit of a pose. Stability is more concerned with muscle contraction to keep the pose strong and stable. For instance, if you were in a downward dog and I come to push you and you fall over, you are not stable so maybe you were using the mobility in your joints to hold the pose rather than muscles. However, in the same case, if you did not fall over then you would be considered to be stable.

Flexibility is the range of motion you have in a muscle i.e., you can do full splits then your muscles and joints have flexibility. However, can you do it without using your hands i.e., use your muscles to take you into the pose. To go into splits pose without hands requires muscle mobility and strength.

Chapter 4
Dialogue

Verbal instructions

Dialogue refers to the words we say in class i.e., verbal instructions. Dialogue is very important because what we say affects what students do.

I have found in all my years teaching that many teacher-training courses don't tend to focus so much on the details of the words, which are used. Most of the time the focus is on the pose, what it looks like and how to do it. Don't misunderstand me it is very important you know the ins and outs of a pose but if you have never taught before then how do you know what to say. You know how to do a pose or what it looks like but when it comes to articulating how to do it, people realise it's actually quite difficult. So where do we get the words from, how do we know what to say? Some courses might offer you dialogue or script and that's a great basis to start to learn how to teach, this tends to happen on courses where the sequence is fixed and it's more of a hot yoga style training it has more static poses rather than a flow style class. The script is a great starting point for sure but months or years down the line this basic script should change especially as you grow as a teacher.

Of course, with most courses, there is a requirement that people have to attend a certain number of classes or practice yoga for a period of time. Now although people attend yoga classes, they do the poses, teaching is a very different idea and quite often people don't realise that until they attend a teacher-training course about how challenging teaching is. Don't get me wrong, after years of teaching it's not difficult anymore but at first, it is and if you change the situation and I was to go teach a large group of students in another part of the world there is a part of me that might get a little nervous, nerves are a sign that you care about what you do so it's a good thing to feel nervous.

Many people who come to training who have to public speak in their job for instance school teachers, who you would expect to excel at public speaking, find it just as hard as those that have never spoken in public. Because this is different and if it's something you are passionate about and it's new and you are outside of your comfort zone.

If you are a banker, you can talk about money and finance all day long with ease as that is what you have done for maybe years, however, that does not mean that you are good at public speaking about everything. If you asked me to talk about finance, I would not have a clue. So the idea of a script is a great idea as it takes away some of the basic worries of how do I say that. You have the words to say and if you say those words, then you can get through the class.

So why does it matter what we say?

Our words guide people in and out of postures, if we say something wrong there is a chance someone will set up the pose incorrectly and they might not be in good alignment. If you have spent years working in finance, it's not very often you will talk about elbows or bending the knees, now, of course, this is a simple language and if English is your first language then these words are easy right? Not necessarily true, if you don't tend to use these words in daily life they might not be that familiar so they can often get mixed up. So why do our verbal instructions matter so much, we can just show a pose?

We are not always able to demonstrate a pose there could be many reasons, please refer to the demonstration section to see why. However, know that dialogue is very important, as it's how we direct people to move into and out of a posture.

With the correct dialogue, we are able to correct many students rather than just one with a hands-on adjustment. What's important about dialogue is that it's clear to the students what we want them to do. The idea being you should be able to teach a blind person using just words only. The way we express instructions can have a negative or positive effect on what we want to achieve so let's just start with the basics i.e., what words we need to say. It is important that when we give instructions they are clear and concise. There are four main dialogue elements to teaching a pose:

1. Person or pose set up dialogue.
2. In posture dialogue.
3. Finisher – The end of a pose.
4. Exit dialogue.

So how do we know where to start when teaching a pose? The first thing you need to consider is what is the purpose of the pose. Understanding the purpose of the pose will help you understand what to cue.

There are of course many variations of poses and depending on the variation depends on what the focus is. So choose the variation you want and know what you want to achieve.

I.e. the focus is leg strength. Of course, different bodies feel things in different ways but if you choose a posture that is focused on leg strength and someone says they feel their back, maybe something is wrong. So you need to look at what went wrong, was the set correct? Do they have good alignment? Is there a postural issue? Or are they meant to feel their back as well as their legs? If that's the case, then was the feeling a good sensation or a bad sensation. Many students say they feel something and you need to establish, is it a muscle pain? It's painful because they are weak or is it the wrong sort of pain?

You should also do the pose yourself, in order to teach something you should try it, test it out where you feel it, how easy is it for you and how difficult was it for you to achieve it. Play with adjustments of your body in the pose i.e., bend the knee more or less, tilt the pelvis slightly, and lift the chest. This is why personal practice is so important you get to feel how small adjustments can affect the pose.

It's good to announce the posture names if you know them. Then, experienced students will know what to do. But keep it simple, "Next is xx pose rather than next we are gonna do…xx pose." Simple instructions are more effective. Does it matter if you don't know the name? No, not really so then just teach and tell them how to get into the pose.

Person or pose set up dialogue

Set-up dialogue is the verbal instructions you use to move people into poses. In most poses, you will move from the anatomical position into the pose. So you need to give exact instructions on how to get into the pose. I often tell students, imagine you're teaching a blind person or even a child that does not know the pose tell them exactly what to do in detail. Although with experienced students, you might be able to get away with saying downward facing dog, for someone who has never done yoga before, they won't even know what it is so lots of detailed instructions are required. The more detail the better because even experienced students may hear some words and adjust their pose.

In posture dialogue

Once you have students in the pose you need to keep them there for a certain amount of time so rather than just saying nothing we have the in-posture dialogue, this dialogue would help them improve their alignment with small adjustments based on your words. This is the best time to encourage people to examine their own poses and improve their alignment.

Finisher – The end of a pose

Towards the end of the pose, students will start to get tired so this is the time when you want to push them to give that little bit more go to their full expression of the pose. Sometimes, students will hold off going to the deepest or full expression if they know they need to hold it for a while but once it's almost at the end, this is the time to push so let them know it's the end and push them with our finisher dialogue.

There are many ways to indicate it is about to end here are just a few:

- Last 10 seconds.
- Last few seconds.
- Go to your maximum.
- Last two breaths.
- Go to your full expression of the pose.

So once you have warned them it's about to end, it's the last chance to push them.

Exit dialogue

This dialogue is simply the words you say to state that the pose has finished. To end the pose, be clear with what you say:

- Change – this is strong. It is used a lot in hot yoga it is obvious something different is happening.
- Release – this works to maybe not as strong as sometimes in a more relaxing pose we will say release down into the pose.
- Come back up.

To finish a pose, you should always close a pose the same way you started. That way, the whole class starts from the same start position so you know you are set up for success. You might simply say feet together arms down by your sides.

Power words vs. powerless words

So what are power words and powerless words? Power words are words that emphasise the action, i.e., lift or reach or stretch. They tend to be short, strong words that are commanding and not vague. Powerless words would be things like bring or spiral. You want to cue the action rather than describe it with some fancy words. It's important that we communicate instructions clearly and concisely so we need to find the most effective way to achieve this. The best way to do this is to be clear, concise and correct. More examples of powerless words or cues will follow.

Powerless words – Examples

Try to – This is okay but today I am tired I don't want to try. If you say, "Try to lift your heels up" or "lift your heels up." The latter is more commanding, it's more of an instruction, and try to give the student the option to not do it. I tried but I can't, or I don't want to try today.

Bring – This is a very common word to use, "bring your arms up," or "bring your leg up." Nothing wrong with it as such but, how about cueing the action.

"Lift your arms up," "reach your arms up," and "stretch your arms up" – These are more effective.

Bring meaning – to come to a place, to carry something with you i.e., please bring a bottle of wine to the party. Julie brought the dog home from the vet.

I also find you cue the action you can put emphasis on the action word i.e., "reach your arms up!" It helps create more lift or more reach.

I want you to – Remember it's not about you it's about the students. So tell them what to do not what you want.

We're gonna – They are doing it not the teacher so yes we could replace this with your gonna but which one sounds better, "you're gonna lift your heels up" or "lift your heels up."

As a teacher, we need to talk a lot so limit words that you don't need to include. The second one also sounds more commanding.

Sorry – This is an interesting word we use in class, often when we make a mistake. It's fine to use it, however, it brings attention to the mistake we made so maybe consider using, "excuse me." It often takes away the feeling of a mistake being made. As we use excuse me when we cough or sneeze or something like that.

Perfect, excellent, good job – These are all great things to say but we have to be careful of overuse. If we say something and a student does it and we say perfect every time, then the word loses its power. So use them to encourage students but not all the time.

Power words – Examples

Power words are simple; cue the action that is happening, examples are:

- Lift.
- Reach.
- Stretch.
- Bend.
- Lengthen.

These are actions words that express the actual action. They are short, strong and commanding.

Types of cues

Artistic/imaginary cues

These types of cues would be used when you want someone to understand the cue. Everyone learns in different ways and some are more visual students and therefore can maybe understand the action with an artistic or imagery cue. Some examples of these would be:

For lateral flexion, for example.

- Paint a rainbow.
- Dial from the ribs.
- Create a half-moon shape.

They all indicate that there will be a specific shape to the body. So these are good for maybe half-moon or gate pose.

If you then wanted to make sure the shoulders were in one line, you could say:

- Imagine your body in between two panes of glass.
- Imagine you are in a toaster.

To open the chest you might say:
- Shine your heart.
- Show your diamond necklace.
- Broaden the collarbone.
- Open your heart.

I would always suggest starting with the basic cue and maybe adding these types of cues in not everyone fully gets it.

Anatomical cues

These types of cues are good for students who have more of an understanding of the body. So it helps them understand what they should feel. If you were in a forward bend, you could say feel your hamstrings stretching. Or even reach the sit bones back to feel your hamstrings more. Sometimes cueing the bones can help people feel it more. You can also use body action cues to help people engage the correct muscle group i.e., press down through the heels to feel the hamstrings. Tilt the pelvis forward and reach the sit bones back. Or simply feel the hamstrings lengthening.

General dialogue

As yoga teachers, we sometimes feel we need to be creative with our language as well as our poses. If we say fancy words, then that makes us sound spiritual or that we are a super teacher. Reality check, simple instructions work best. Most people are in their own world and don't listen and in reality, they want to walk out of that room feeling different and no matter how many super fancy words you say, it's the practice that will make them feel different.

When teaching, you want to ensure you cue all the main key actions and make it concise.

Sometimes, we need to shorten the cues take out the nice flowery stuff and just cue action. If a student were to listen to a recording of the instructor speaking the instructions, are the cues were clear and concise enough such that the student could follow along with the recording without confusion.

It's very nice to say spiral your thighs inwards or open your heart to grace but maybe something like knees together or shoulders back might also be easier to understand.

So how do we structure our dialogue you need to think?

Verb + Body part + Direction.

"Lift heels up." That's a verb, body part and direction but it sounds too robotic and there is no ownership of the cue.

"Lift your heels up." Works better because it means there is ownership and each instruction is clear.

I have often heard things like:

1. "Lift your heels up for me."
2. "Let's lift our heels up."
3. "Your heels are lifting."
4. "Lift those heels up."
5. "Lift these heels up."
6. "Lift that heel up."

So let's look at why these are not the best cues, they are not wrong as such there are just better ways we can say them. So let's look at why some of these don't work so well.

- The students are not practising for the benefit of you the teacher; they come for their own practice. We guide them but essentially the class is for them, not us. So, therefore, saying do this for me means the class becomes about us the teacher and not the students.
- You, the teacher, are not practising so it should never be, we or us.
- Use more commanding verbs rather than passive ones, saying what your heels need to do rather than what they are doing. By adding the -'ing', it makes it more passive like you're describing what someone is doing rather than telling them what they need to do. This is more like storytelling.
- 4–6 are the same, make sure the students have ownership of their practice, it should be, lift your heels up. If you say that, those, them, and then which heels are you referring to, her heels or his heels. If you say that knee, which one is the left knee or the right knee.

Lock your (knees/elbows)

This is always a very controversial subject. Lock your knees or lock your elbows has been a cue often heard in hot yoga classes. So am I suggesting it's wrong, yes and no? In essence, what students understand from it the cue is wrong however the original source from where it came it's not wrong but ensuring students understand that is complicated especially in a group class situation. Yoga in India was mainly taught one-on-one so it would have been easy to ensure students understood this cue but in a large group class, it's often misunderstood.

So let's first look at the origin or what it means. The original name that was used for the knee lock was called 'Janu Bandha', which is a knee lock. The lock refers to a co-contraction of all opposing muscles surrounding the joint complex. That means a number of muscles should be contacted such as quadriceps, hamstrings, calf muscles, adductors and abductors etc. should all contract to stabilise the knee joint. Over time, the phrase, lock the knee has taken on another meaning, which basically means the leg should be perfectly straight. Which in the case of some people is fine but for those that have hypermobility of the knee joint means that they would hyperextend the knee.

So what is hyperextension and what does it mean? When the leg is perfectly straight, the lateral malleolus (ankle bone) is in line with the greater trochanter (hip bone) and Lateral epicondyle (knee bone). If the knee is hyperextended, it means that the knee bone will be behind the ankle and hipbone. Is this bad? Not necessarily some people have flexible joints naturally and for some, it's due to weakness or an over-stretched muscle.

So how do we prevent hyperextension? We need to strengthen the muscle group which flexes the knee joint, the hamstrings. You might hear a teacher say, lift the quadriceps, up but the quadriceps is in the front of the leg and won't help prevent the knee joint from going back it will, in fact, encourage it. So, you need to work on the posterior leg muscle strength, hence it's the hamstring. But does it really matter if a person who has super flexible joints locks the joint? Everyone is different in their structure and make-up, someone who has flexible joints might experience no issues or no pain ever in their life. Some might experience pain, as they may overstretch ligaments around the joints. For those that don't experience pain ever, does it matter? Yes, it does because what it means is they are not using muscles to move or stabilise the joint. The idea is to strengthen muscles as muscles move the joints so although they may have no pain it means that they are relying on ligaments to stabilise the joint. Joints should be moved using muscles, not force or ligaments.

In order to teach yoga, you should know a bit about anatomy. There are many reasons why you would need to know at least a basic anatomy. Understanding anatomy helps you understand how to give verbal instructions on how to get into a pose.

1. You need to know what muscles are being affected by the pose.
2. How are they being affected, i.e., stretched or strengthened.
3. If someone has an injury or tightness, you need to know how to modify the pose.
4. You need to know where in the body students should be feeling a pose and why some find it harder than others.

When we talk about what is happening in terms of anatomy, we always start from the anatomical position. See below for anatomical position, this would be the start position and we would move into poses from this position. Your instructions should be clear and easy to understand.

So, what is anatomical position, the body is standing upright, with the feet at shoulder width and parallel, toes forward. The upper limbs are held out to each side, and the palms of the hands face forward. This is the start position and in yoga, we often refer to this as the mountain pose. From here, we move into a pose. So what do we need to know about a pose?

1. The purpose of the pose, what is our goal with this pose today? Some poses have many factors i.e., open hips and strengthen the legs but what is the focus for today? For instance, in warrior 2 the focus is to open the hips or strengthen the legs. Maybe it's both in that case your cues need to reflect both possibilities.
2. What parts of the body need to move to achieve that, movement comes from the joints so you need to know what joints need to move in what way in order to achieve the pose. In the case of warrior 2, if the hip needs to externally rotate then what do we need to say to achieve that. Cue how wide the step is, and where should the knee be in order to be safe. Should the thigh be parallel if so, cue that. All the cues should be easily understandable by students and don't assume that experienced students know what they are doing it is possible they have done it wrong and someone has not corrected them.
3. Why will some students find it more challenging than others, our bodies are different, bone structure,

muscle structure, and history in terms of injuries or habits. So no two people will look or feel the same exact same thing. A cyclist will have strong quadriceps and might not feel their quads so much but might feel their gluteus. Even though people's bodies are different as long as we cue correctly, we know everyone is safe and differences may be due to weakness or tightness or simply posture.

4. What is likely to restrict someone doing the pose, is it muscle tightness, weakness, ligament tightness, fascia, bone structure, and short or long limbs? So many factors. Impossible to decipher which ones during a group class situation but as long as everyone is set up correctly you know they are safe and maybe you can talk directly with specific students after class to help them further.
5. How should we modify a pose for someone? You need to understand why someone needs a modification. Is it because they can't do the pose, or what if they experience pain in the pose? If you know what is the essence of a pose i.e., hamstring stretching it's easier to find a modification.
6. If someone has a specific, injury can they do that pose? They recently had knee surgery can they kneel? They hurt their knee skiing can they fully flex the knee. These are things we need to think about.

All of a sudden teaching yoga now sounds difficult, but it's not if you know as much as you can about a pose and follow some simple rules. So in order to understand what happens in a pose, we need to understand movement, where it comes from, how people compensate etc. So let's look at awkward poses and what happens in general and then in detail.

Awkward pose

When we think of an awkward pose, it is a pretty simple pose, so not too complicated, or so we think. There are a number of variations of this pose but for the purpose of this example, I will refer to the hot yoga style version part 1.

Awkward part 1 – General
- Hips and knees are flexed, feet hips distance apart.
- Ankles Dorsi flexed.
- Spine is in slight extension or neutral.
- Shoulders are flexed and slightly internally rotated and elbows are pronated.

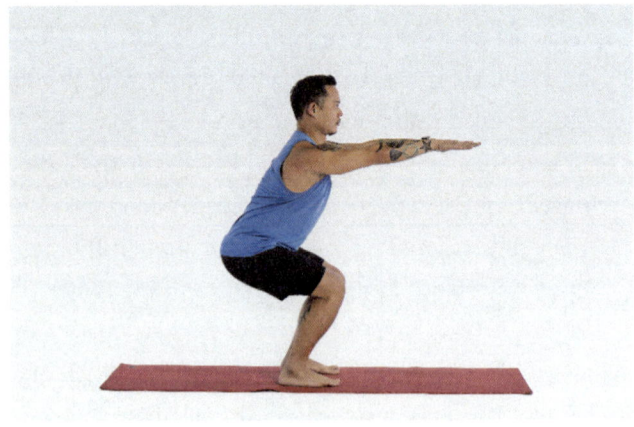

Awkward

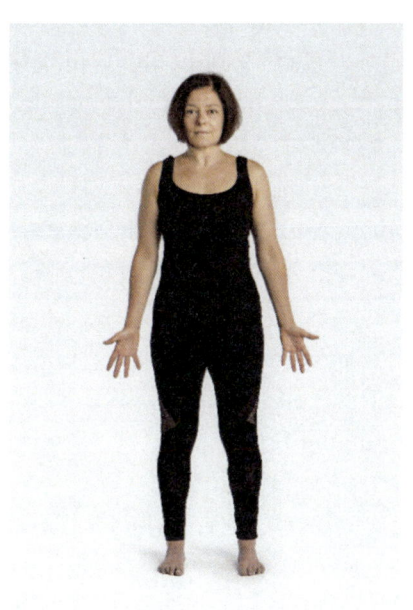

Anatomical Position

So in detail, we need to know how to create that movement i.e., how to flex the hips and know what muscle makes the movement and what restricts the movement. The best way to think of set-up is to think from the ground up, the ground is where you should start and then move up the body. Now, once you understand the essence of the posture you should know what to cue and what needs to be corrected. The main focus of this pose is leg strength and mobility of the hips knees and ankles. So set that up correctly.

So let's break these down further.

Set up is important but why? It's our job as teachers to ensure students are safe and they don't hurt themselves. So the start position is key, "Set up for success."

Feet hips distance apart

Start at the base where should the feet be, they should be hips distance apart so you need to make that the first action.

Two possible cues are:

- 'Separate your feet hips distance apart'.
- 'Step the right foot to the right'.

So let's examine each cue as one is more appropriate for a large group and the other might work for a smaller group, neither is wrong though.

- ***Separate your feet hips distance apart*** – This can be hips distance, or 15 cm, or six inches as long as the cue works with the audience i.e., they know what 15 cm is. Ideally, you want people with their feet at hips to distance apart according to their body, bearing in mind everyone had a different-sized pelvis and hips. Although it is also true, some people don't know how big their hips are so some teachers' cue two fists distance between the feet, which also works.

So how about cue number 2

- ***Step your right foot to the right*** – have you ever wondered why people don't just say open your feet? By the whole class stepping to the right, it should mean that most students could still see themselves in the mirror. Once you have said this, you should clarify with feet, hips distance apart.

Now we have the position of the feet and how should they be. Turn out, parallel, turn in. In the case of this pose, they should be parallel.

Feet parallel

So here are some cues:

- 'Looks like the number 11'.
- 'Toes in heels out'.
- 'Second toe points forward'.

This is a simple movement but has lots of considerations and things to think about. The cues above should suffice on a basic teaching level but there are some things as a teacher that you should know to help to understand why sometimes feet parallel is hard. There is a tendency that people will not have their feet exactly parallel this is because we walk, and we tend to have a slight turnout. So, to put your feet exactly parallel can feel very odd and so, as humans we tend to lean towards comfort rather than discomfort. However, if the pose requires to feel parallel then that's what we need to encourage students to aim for. The position of the feet can affect other joints further up the leg. If the feet are lined up correctly, then the pelvis will be correctly aligned. Feet parallel means that the second toe should line up with the middle of the ankle when the feet are parallel so you should see a straight line if you were to continue that line forward. This makes sure we activate the adductor and abductors equally and ensures no torque on the knees.

I hear some teachers talk about the inside edge of the foot or the outside edge of the foot being parallel. This would largely depend on the foot shape, as everyone is slightly different, for me if I line the outside edge of the foot parallel to the mat it makes me turn my thighs inwards, which is not correct.

When doing standing poses, the base needs to be strong and stable i.e., you need to ensure you press three corners of the foot down, big toe little toe and evenly on the heel. Due to habits or muscle imbalances, students will press more weight on the big toe or the little toe. The weight might favour the outside of the foot or the inside. You have to consider the focus of the pose is to keep the hips neutral, if so, then the feet should be parallel.

One thing to consider is exact parallel feet can also be hard to achieve according to the shape of your pelvis and how your hip sockets are placed. If your hip sockets face more lateral, then it is likely you have more mobility in lateral rotation but might mean that when you are in neutral, your feet might not be parallel. Of course, this is not something you can check just by looking. You need to get the student to engage all the leg muscles to lift the arches of the foot. Once this is done place the feet in parallel if the knees turn in there is a good chance that the hip sockets are more lateral so in order to achieve this foot position they actually need to internally rotate the femur bone, which would be incorrect.

Of course, we can't manage the situation for each and every student who has a different body but it's our job to have as much information as we can in order to help students practice with the correct posture according to their body. For a large group situation, you would just say feet parallel. For a private or small group, there is more chance that you can adjust people individually. If you have a student that you suspect might have an issue with feet parallel, you can always talk to them directly after class. If someone does have more lateral rotation in their hips and in order to place their feet in parallel, they need to internally rotate their femur bones in, does it matter? It will give them more space across their lumbar spine so it might feel good but if their knees fall in and they experience pain then that's not good. The most important factor is everyone is safe; remember that in managing a large group, it's impossible to get everyone to do the right thing all the time. Actually, the 'normal' position for the feet is a five-degree turnout.

So now we have the feet sorted what's next, well you would think hips maybe as we move up the body. But when we go to sit down we go backwards slightly so we need a counterbalance, the next part is the arms.

Arms up

Should the arms be shoulder-level? Yes, they should so then we should say arms up in line with the shoulders, or shoulder level. A basic instruction arms up shoulder level will get the result you want for sure. Students will tend to do one of two things, i.e., not lift high enough or lift too high that they elevate their shoulders.

In order to refine this, you can add in:

- 'Shoulder blades down, or slide the shoulders down'.

The deltoids work hard in order to keep the shoulders in flexion and they often get tired so we need to recruit the biceps and triceps to support the deltoids. Telling students to engage their biceps when their arms are straight can be an impossible instruction for students to understand, i.e., how can I engage an elbow flexor muscle when my elbow is extended? So the best way to cue one of the following:

- 'Strong arms'.
- 'Reach the fingers forward'.
- 'Keep reaching your arms long'.

This idea of reaching can help contract the muscles we need to recruit. However, sometimes number two and three can often lead to the protraction of the scapula (shoulder blades separate at the back) because they reach too far forward. We want to keep a neutral position of the scapula so we need to ensure they are neutral in terms of the back and front. In this pose, the spine is either neutral or slight extension. Protraction helps facilitate spinal flexion this means that a protracted scapula would be incorrect for this pose.

Cueing to 'slide shoulder blades back or broaden the collar bone' should help fix this.

We have to consider what the purpose of this pose is, the main focus is not to strengthen the shoulders the main focus is hip and knee mobility along with leg strength. The arms help as a counterbalance for the hips going back.

Sit down

- 'Bend your knees, hips down'.
- 'Sit down as if you are sitting down in a chair'.

How far should they bend their knees, and how low should they sit?

- Should the knees be in line with the hips?
- Should the hips be higher than the knees?
- Knees higher than the hips?

- Knees in line with hips.

This is ideal but it can't always be achieved as it's the goal. Sometimes students don't sit down low enough because it's hard, maybe they are not strong. If this is the case, we encourage them each time to go further in order to build strength. Sometimes it can be a tightness in muscles, again we could encourage them to sit down and keep working at it each time they practice. There might be other reasons such as bone structure, which can prevent someone from sitting lower, we will address that point later on.

- Knees higher than hips.

Let's consider what happens if the hips are lower than the knees, once the hips go low, we are able to sit more into the joints and the quads will be less active, this means that you are not getting the same strength in your legs. It also means the initial point of lifting backup is going to be hard as you need to activate your quads again. So what students tend to do is lift up quickly without control. There is a flexibility benefit of course but if you want to build strength, it won't be as much.

- Hips higher than knees.

This often means someone has not sat down low enough, although the hips might be slightly higher this is okay but if like in the picture it's either weakness or a student has taken the easy option. So we encourage them to sit lower.

The ideal position is to keep the hips slightly higher or at the same level as the knees.

Pelvis

Let's talk about the pelvis. The position of the pelvis is also very important; ideally, we want the pelvis to remain neutral, with maybe a slight anterior tilt. In the original pose, the spine was neutral so the pelvis would be neutral. With the current lifestyle, we lead we spend much more time sitting, which leads to tighter hip flexors, which can exaggerate an anterior pelvic tilt. If the hips flexors are tight when we squat down, we often find that the lumbar extends more and we get an exaggerated anterior tilt. Teachers will often cue tuck the tailbone under or scoop the tailbone, this is one cue that I personally don't like. The reason I don't like this cue is for these reasons:

- The position of the pelvis should be neutral and not a posterior pelvic tilt by tucking the tailbone under this can create a posterior pelvic tilt. Imagine if someone already naturally has a posterior pelvic tilt they will hear this cue and tuck even more. This can also then create a rounding of the upper back i.e., thoracic flexion, which is also not ideal for this pose. This is where sometimes we need to be careful with cues for someone who does have an anterior tilt or extremely extended lumbar spine like me saying tucking the tailbone might get me to the right position but like as mentioned above it can cause others to be in the wrong set up.

Better cues for group class would be:

- 'Point the tailbone down'.
- 'Lengthen the lower back'.

Awkward – In posture dialogue

So that's the posture set-up, next we need to give them the 'in-posture dialogue' cues. So whilst students are holding a pose we have options.

We can just count, inhale for five, inhale for four but counting does not help students improve their posture it just indicates the time left until we change to something else. So, it's better to cue some alignment corrections so they can improve their posture. You can still count of course but maybe rather than say four after three, maybe give a constructive cue.

Even if you have given all the correct instructions to start with, this does not always mean students have the correct alignment. Some don't listen, some don't understand what the cues mean, and some will think they have feet parallel but they don't. For some, it's just too hard so they take the easy option which might not be correct. Our minds can often drift off when we are in yoga, especially for those who know what to do, it's like we know what to do so we just do it without thinking. There are many reasons why students do not have the correct alignment.

So we can now take time whilst they are in the pose to correct them. New students are great in this situation because the chances are they did not do the pose correctly so you are able to look at them and correct them verbally by saying certain cues, which of course the whole group will hear and benefit from. Furthermore, as our body gets tired in a pose, we tend to lose focus and this will often lead to misalignments. The one thing for sure is you cannot repeat instructions enough. Sometimes we lose focus and maybe we don't hear an instruction or maybe we did not understand so repeating gives the student the chance to hear the instruction again.

So what often goes wrong in this pose?

1. As they sit down, they turn their feet out.
2. Their knees go forward of the ankles.
3. They don't sit low enough.
4. They sit too low.
5. Their feet are too narrow or too wide.
6. Their toes come off the mat.
7. They lower their arms.
8. They lean the body forward in order to go deeper.
9. They over arch their lower back.

How do we fix these issues and in which order? You can look around a room and see so many things gone wrong and it can be daunting, how do I fix all this with all these students? That's where the power of your words comes into play.

When students do things wrong, it gives you the perfect time to say some corrective dialogue. So which ones do we correct first, well it depends on what you think is the focus for the class, plus also consider which option they are likely to injure their body. The general idea is to go from the ground up. So feet, knees, hips, torso, arms, head etc. but consider also what could go wrong.

Lowering their arms is often due to weakness, they won't hurt themselves but knees going forward of ankles can put too much load on the knees as its harder to engage the glutes and hanstrings and the focus is on the quadriceps. So order your instructions i.e., which one first. Our set-up instructions start at the feet so we should follow this order so we know we have covered it all.

Let's look at how we can cue them to correct them and also look at why this might happen.

1. As they sit down, they turn their feet out.

Possible Cues:

- o 'Toes in. heels out'.
- o 'Look at your feet and make sure they are parallel'.

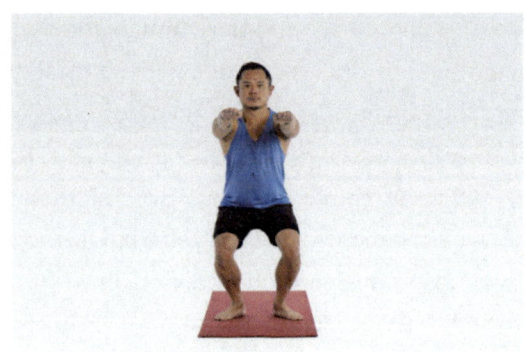

Awkward

Why did this happen?

- This is the easier option if people are very open in the hips they will naturally lean towards more of a turn in our position.
- It makes it easier to balance as the base is wider.

2. Their knees go forward of the ankles

- o 'Weight in the heels'.
- o 'Send the bum back, not the knees forward'.
- o 'Look down at your feet and check you can see your toes'.

Why did this happen?

- You use less Hamstrings and gluteus, so it's easier to push the knees forward.

- Their ankles are super mobile and people don't know they do it wrong.

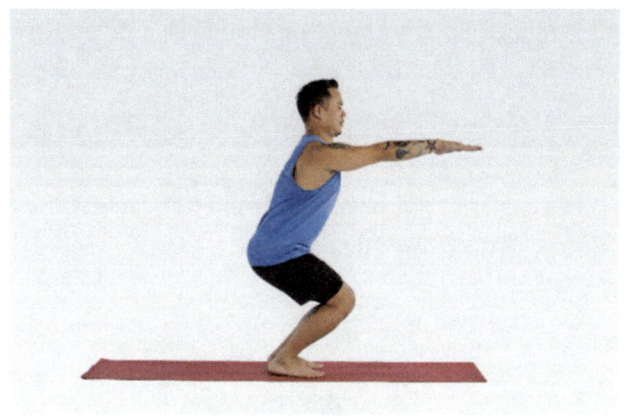

Awkward

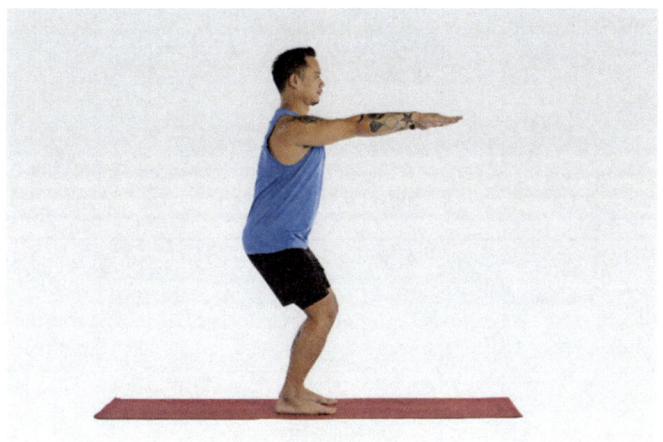

Awkward

3. They don't sit low enough

- o   'Sit down deeper'.
- o   'Thighs parallel to the floor'.

Why did they not sit low enough?

- It's easier to not have knees and hips in line.
- Maybe they can't due to tight ankles.

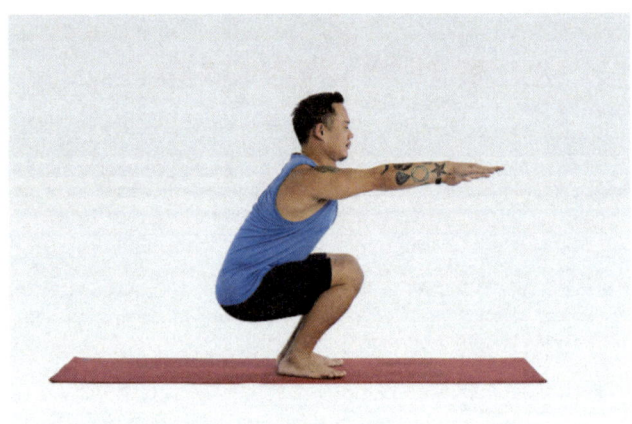

Awkward

4. They sit too low

- o 'Hips should be higher than the knees'.
- o 'If there were a ball on your knees, it would roll off'.

Why do they sit too low?

- The teacher told them to sit low and be the smallest person in the room.
- It's easier to sit lower the quads don't work as hard.
- They think they are doing their posture better by sitting lower, but they are not.

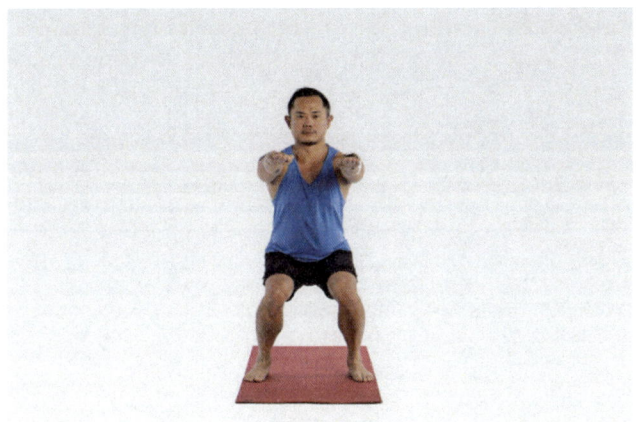

Awkward

5. Their feet are too narrow or too wide

- o 'Keep your feet in line with your hips'.
- o 'Equal distance between feet, knees and arms'.
- o 'Equal weight on inside and outside edge of the foot'.
- o 'Knees in line with ankles'.

Why does this happen?

- People don't know how big their hips are.
- Most assume their hips are smaller than they think.
- People go wider because it's a bigger base so more stability.

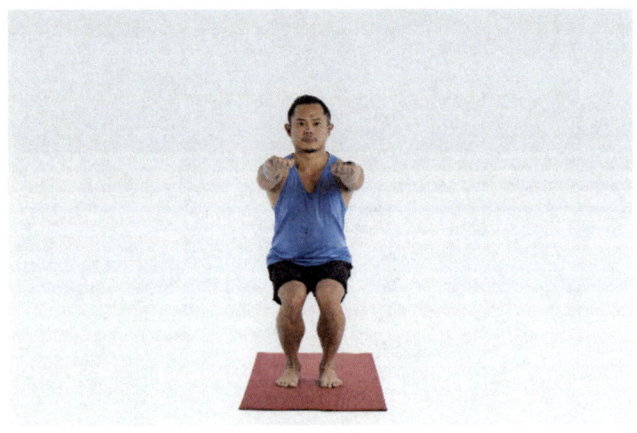

Awkward

6. Their toes off the mat

o   'Press the toes softly into the mat'.
o   'Press the weight back into the heels with the toes down'.

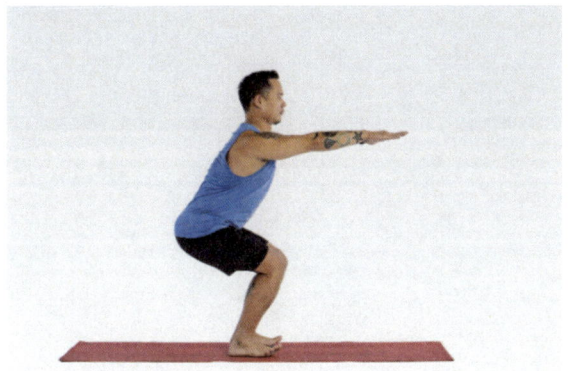

Awkward

Why does this happen?

- This tends to happen when our cue weight is in the heels people check by lifting their toes up. This creates added tension to the shinbones and over-activates the ankle flexor muscles.
- They don't know how to push the weight back.

7. They lower their arms

- 'Strong arms'.
- 'Keep the arms in line with the shoulders'.
- 'Reach the arms long to help engage the biceps and triceps'.

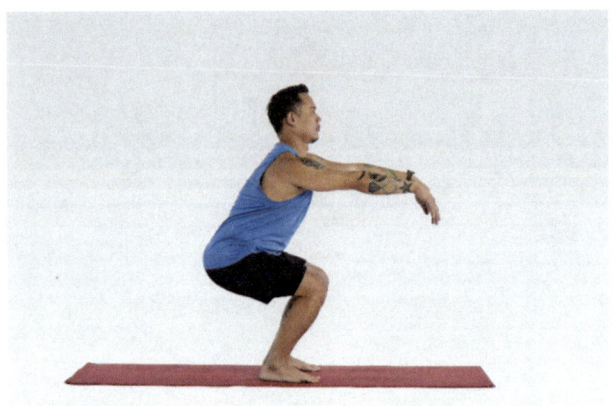

Awkward

Why does this happen?

- They often lower their arms because they overuse deltoids so encourage them to engage their biceps and triceps to support their deltoids.
- They get tired.

8. They lean their upper body forward to go deeper.

o   'Lift your chest up'.
o   'Lean the upper body back'.

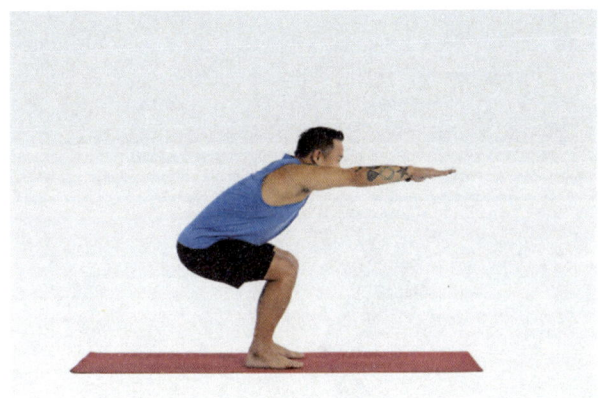

Awkward

Why does this happen?

- Tight hip flexors pull the body forward.
- Student tries to go deeper but can't so they lean forward.
- Core not engaged.
- Weak gluteus.
- Leaning forward can put added pressure on the lower back and knees and often means less gluteus engagement.

9. They over arch their lower back

- o 'Lengthen the lower back'.
- o 'Point the tailbone down'.
- o 'Engage your abs'.

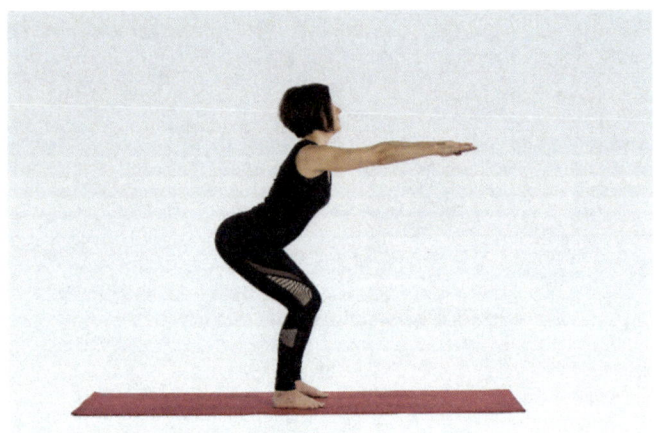

Awkward

Why does this happen?

- Hip flexors are tight when they lift the chest the back goes into further extension.
- It's easier for people with mobile lumbar spines to sink into the lower back.
- When your lower back arches, the gluteus tends to switch off; they are big muscles so we should use them.

- This means the abs are not engaged are supporting the back, maybe the abs are weak or the back muscles are too strong.

So the cues above are corrective cues, to correct alignment issues. How about other types of cues like where to feel it, what muscles to feel and small corrections to feel muscles more. So let's examine what is going on in the posture.

Hips flexed – What muscles flex the hips

Hip flexors – The hip flexors are made up of a number of muscles most obvious are the Iliacus and Psoas Major, also two thigh muscles also help that is the Rectus femoris and Sartorius. Of course, you would not necessarily spout off all the muscles in class but knowing it is key and you can say feel your hip flexors and indicate where they are. It's also important to know the anatomy of poses so that you can help modify them when someone has an injury. It's important to know that some students will feel things in different areas due to weaknesses and strengths. Quite often, big muscles take over.

The Psoas originates at the lumbar spine and attaches to the femur bone; it's the only muscle that connects the upper body with the lower body. If it's tight, it can pull on the lower back and can cause lower back pain. In an awkward pose, the spine is in a slight extension or neutral, but you need to be careful as people with tight hip flexors may over-extend the lumbar spine.

Knees flexed

The hamstrings flex the knees and often people with tight hamstrings often struggle to fully extend the knee to the neutral. So what restricts knee flexion is the quadriceps, if they are tight someone will find it hard to fully flex the knee, i.e., move the heel to the hip. This pose requires only 90 degrees of knee flexion and most people should be able to achieve this without any issues though.

Feet hips distance apart

Knees in line with feet should be straightforward but it's not. If your adductors are tight, they will pull the knees inwards. If the abductors are weak, they will push the knees inwards and holding them out will be harder. External rotator weakness can also cause the knees to fall inwards.

Shoulders are flexed and internally rotated

Shoulder flexion is limited by your shoulder flexor muscles, i.e., Latissimus Dorsi, and Teres Major. If they are tight, they will limit the range of motion but in this pose, only 90 degrees of flexion is required so it's very unlikely there will be restrictions at this level. Internal rotation comes from the Pecs, Subscapularis and latissimus Dorsi. This is again not a full range of motion so is unlikely to be restricted.

Ankles dorsiflexed

Ankle mobility will restrict how far someone can sit down. This can be due to tight calf muscles, Gastrocnemius or Soleus; another possibility is a tight Achilles tendon. If it's due to tight muscles, then stretching the tight muscles will help increase the range of motion.

Another possibility is bone compression i.e., bone hits bone if this is the case there is nothing that can be done. There are tests that can be done to assess to see if it's bone on bone. Often students won't complain of tightness they will simply say, I just can't go any further. As a teacher, you are not expected to be able to assess this however notice things like, how far they sit down in part 1 and then how far they sit down in part 2. The main difference is the angle of the ankle joint, which changes when you lift your heels up. The normal range of motion or dorsi flexion is 20 degrees and 50 degrees for plantar flexion.

The other consideration is why some students cannot do this, why they don't look quite right what is restricting them.

1. Tight muscles will restrict people but over time this can change. You need to stretch and strengthen tight muscles. Also, consider the opposing group and make sure you work with them equally too as both sides should be balanced.
2. Bone structure – cannot be changed, when bone hits bone it is called compression so nothing you can do to change this so modify as required.
3. Short or long limbs can make someone look different or find certain poses more challenging i.e., it's harder to bind in a pose you have short arms, or hard to lift up if you can't reach the floor. This is where yoga props are useful.
4. Joint mobility, it could simply just be tightness of the joint, not bones or muscles, maybe ligaments or other

tissues. So stretching and mobilising the joint is important. Moving the joint in all directions is key.

Mobility in the hips, ankles and spine plays an important role in this pose. The knees don't go to the full range so it's unlikely tight hamstrings will make a huge difference to how this pose looks. However tight ankles or a tight spine can.

Hip flexors – Will pull the upper body forward, this can put the spine into further hyperextension and will pull the pelvis forward. This can put lots of pressure on the lumbar spine and furthermore, this action can rotate the femur bone inwards and consequently the knees will fall inwards.

Abs/Rectus abdominis – Tight rectus can cause the upper back and the thoracic spine to flex forward, which makes it hard to lean the upper body back. Most will dump into the lumbar spine as it's more mobile in extension.

Tight calf muscles – If the posterior lower leg muscles such as gastrocnemius or soleus are tight the ankle might have limited mobility.

How to give corrective cues

As a teacher, we can cue muscles i.e., engage your quads but although most will know what the quads are, they won't know all the muscles. I find it easier to either cue the bones or cue what body part to be pressing down.

Some people don't actually know how to contract a muscle so rather than say engage x muscle I will give them cues which I know will directly affect a muscle or muscle group. Some examples are below:

Hamstrings

Press down through the heels.

Push the weight back into the heels.

Reach the sit bones. (Sit bones or ischium is the origin of the hamstrings.)

Obliques

Move the ribs closer to the hips.

Rotate from the rib cage keeping the pelvis stable.

Reach the crown of the head up, keep a long spine, and lengthen through the spine Rotate the right shoulder to the left hip.

Side bend to the right, ribcage moves closer to the pelvis.

Scapular muscles

Broaden the collarbone.

Actively press the hands/forearms down.

Press the upper back up and away Create space across the upper back.

Chapter 5
Voice

Why is the voice so important?

The voice is a powerful tool in yoga teaching, with your hands, you can touch only one person at a time but with your voice, you can reach many. How we use our voice is important as our instructions can be delivered to a room of 50 people at one time. So it's important that we take care of our voice and use it wisely. You want to be able to project to the whole room so you can keep your 'audience' or students engaged. Teachers who teach a lot at first can suffer with sore throats and lose their voice so you want to always speak from your chest and find power from your stomach and not your throat so you save your throat from getting sore.

Tone, tempo and rhythm are important. You don't want to talk so fast that students don't even know what you're saying and it feels like you are at a horse race. This is quite common for new teachers, as we get nervous and excited we tend to increase our speed. I was very guilty of this and can still be too fast when I get excited about something. You also want to ensure you don't drag the words so that it feels like a slow death by yoga. These are all skills that you will acquire over time that will help you become a better teacher.

Tone of voice

So now we know roughly what to say, how do we say it and does it matter. The tone of voice can have a huge effect on energy, on how hard a student works, or how they feel in a certain pose. Students and teachers share energy in class so if you want your students to work hard and push themselves then we need to be seen to be giving them all we have. So let's look at a few scenarios to see how this plays out.

Back bending – Let's face it, it's super hard for most people to spine twist. This is more of a cool-down or warm-up pose, which is more relaxing seated forward fold. It's more about stretching, it does not require huge strength to do it. Balancing stick – Short, strong and powerful.

When we look at voice tones, often we think when something is harder we need to get louder this is not always the case. Louder is an option yes but consider, the pitch of the voice. If by getting louder your pitch becomes more 'high-pitched', it does not work. We end up sounding like Mickey Mouse, which does not work if we want to be commanding. In fact, most of the time you want to consider going down a level and having a deeper voice.

Examples of different tones

So what types of tones do we have?
Level 1 – Soft, calm yet clear.
Level 2 – Clear and level.
Level 3 – Strong and rising.

Level 4 – High constant.

So how would we apply these tones to poses?

Level 1 – Spine twist or final relaxation is a good choice for this level. You are not pushing students at this point the focus is release and relaxation so the voice needs to match that. I would call this the 'Spa voice'. Not only should your voice be not so loud, but it's also a good time to say words in a different way by changing where you put the emphasis. The words become longer i.e., 'relaxxxx' so you emphasise the end of the word and the tone goes down towards the end.

Level 2 – Seated forward fold and separate leg stretch is a good choice for this. It's not about pushing. This voice I would call the 'standard voice', it's more how we normally speak. The poses are not hard as such so we don't need to push. Words are clear and no need for a special tone or change of emphasis or a specific part of the word. Just make words clear, tone of voice remains the same level throughout.

Level 3 – Strong and rising. This is the perfect voice for something like a Standing bow pose or a Half moon. A pose where the pose might be held for some time and you need to push at the end. I call this the 'Sports Commentary' voice. It starts at a constant level but you need to raise it towards the end, much like how a football commentator would change his tone as the striker gets nearer to the goal. If a pose is challenging and held longer, then the last part of the pose is important as students just want to quit, but as teachers, we need to encourage them to push a bit further at the end. We have many ways we can push someone at the end:

1. Increase the volume at which you speak, but keep the pitch the same.

2. Increase the speed at which you speak.
3. Shorten the words, making them more commanding.
4. You can also decrease the speed, i.e., short words but they must be strong and commanding.

Level 4 – High constant. This tone we use when we teach short difficult poses, i.e., balancing stick or any backbend. We need students to stay in the pose so we have to give them a reason. I call this voice 'horse race' voice. Horse races are short and fast so it needs to be the same energy throughout. Generally, words are short the pace is faster and possibly louder. Lots of high energy, commanding words and strong.

Could we teach all in the same tone, of course, you could but it's fair to say if you taught all in Level 4 it would be wrong much like all in level 1 would also be wrong. It's good to change the tone of your voice in order to differentiate what you want students to do, i.e., push and work hard, or relax and chill a bit. Changing tone does not mean getting loud; it means making the tone different. There are many ways you can push students:

1. Get louder.
2. Talk slower to hold postures longer.
3. Emphasise certain words, i.e., make them longer like stretchhhhhhhh or Pushhhhh.
4. Shorten the words to more commanding words with pauses to make them stronger, i.e., Lift…your…heels… up… higher.

So that gives us an idea of what types of tones and voices we use within certain poses but what about other times in class, i.e., the set-up of a pose or when we come out of a pose. Having taught in some countries where English is not the first language I have learnt other ways to use my voice to ensure students know something different is going to happen.

Change your tone for certain parts for the class

Pose set up – Should be Level 2. Clear with simple instructions.

Transition voice – should be level 2 in that it's a constant level but more like level 3 in that it's louder, i.e., something different will happen.

There are other times when you need to adjust your voice, for instance, hands to feet pose would be a level 2, you need to be clear and constant however when people have their heads down, i.e., they can't see the teacher it's important that they can hear the teacher clearly so you may need to lift your volume a little to be sure they can hear. In my experience, when people can't see, they can't seem to follow instructions as easily. So a level of 2.5 might be needed here.

Exiting a pose

When you're at the end of a pose, raise your voice to give students that final push. I find it useful to increase volume when something is going to change so that your students know something different is coming. This technique is especially useful if you're teaching students who might not use English as their first language. That way, even if they don't understand what you have said they know something different has happened.

Change your tone for certain classes

Some teachers will have a naturally louder voice or a softer voice. Of course, you should always honour your skills and not try to be something you are not. However, you need to consider the class you are teaching also, for instance, if you were to teach a kickboxing class with a soft gentle tone it would not work. As would teaching a yin class with a strong loud powerful voice. As well as certain poses, certain classes should also have different tones.

Not only would I change my tone of voice for a gentler yin-style class but I would also change how I put emphasis on certain words. Like, stretch or lengthen or artistic words like melt or sink. Phrases such as 'melt like caramel', come to mind it feels yummy and soft and feels like I can let go. I might even include breathing or audio sounds like arhhhh. To help emphasise what I want to happen.

Chapter 6
Body Language

Your own body language whilst teaching

Body language is very important when teaching, we of course can do nothing and just stand against the wall but it does not help students, and indicates to students that we are not interested in want we do. Body language is important because we can use our bodies to help students understand instructions. There are many reasons why students might not understand instructions.

1. You are teaching in a language which is not so familiar to them, i.e., It's their second language.
2. They don't have good body awareness, I see this a lot when students get confused about left and right or elbows and knees.
3. They are simply in their own world or did not hear the instruction.
4. Maybe the instruction was not clear.

Body language also helps when trying to get the student to go further by over exaggerating the movement we can get students to maybe move a little further. So what body language should be avoided and why?

- Hands on hips.
- Hands behind the back.
- Clasping hands in the front.
- Checking out the nails.

Hands on hips

There is no reason to place our hands on our hips other than we don't know what to do with our hands. So why should we not do it:

- Hands on hips will not help us to teach a good class.
- Hands on hips can make the teacher look full of themselves, it can come across are quite stern and unfriendly.

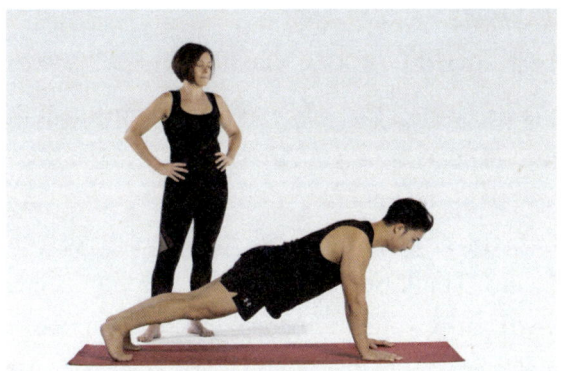

Hands behind the back

It's just not the best thing we can do. Like the one above, it can make you look too commanding and not friendly. If that's what you want to achieve, then go ahead but for me, teaching yoga is about controlling the class with a strong presence but with a friendly face so people know it's a safe space.

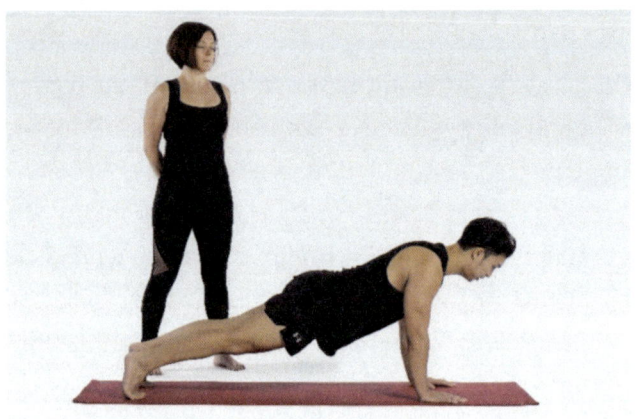

Clasping hands in the front

This is a true sign that someone is not confident. It might be the case especially if you are new to teaching, however, even if you don't feel confident fake it and pretend you do. It requires a very open posture, one that can make you feel a little insecure. Think of it like this: when a lion is coming at you, you will close your body down this is a scared protection position. However, when we are in love, we are very open and our body shows this so it's a much nicer body stance to offer it shows we are open and not closed.

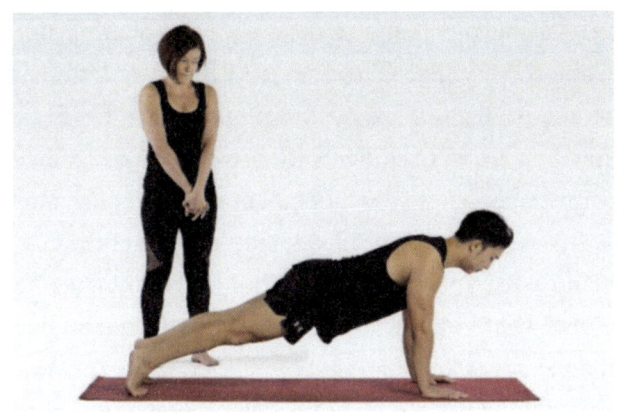

Checking out the nails

This type of pose indicates that you are not really present. I am not 100% here with you I would rather be walking in the park.

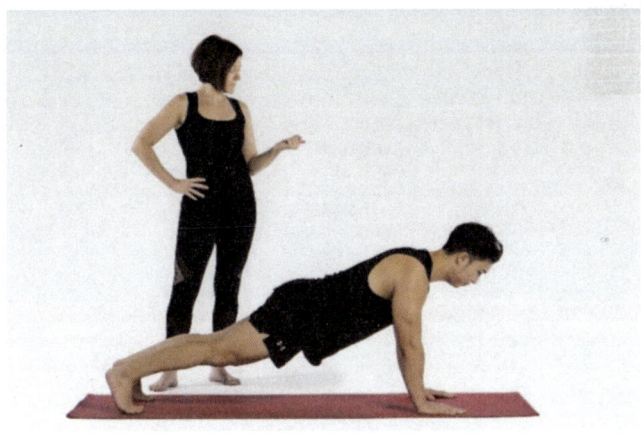

We should use our body to express what we want students to do. By using our body, it shows we are sharing our full energy and they will give back to us. I know as a student if I feel the energy from a teacher trying their best I will do my best. So when we want students to side bend to one side using your arms to emphasise the movement can help push students further. It also helps a lot with students who maybe don't fully understand what you are saying. Your body language should also reflect what you want to achieve if you want students to relax then exaggerate your movements and make them slower and more deliberate. You can do this by reaching your arms forward like you trying to stretch out of your body and adding in the voice like reachhh arhhh, students will feel it. If you want them to work harder, make the movements quicker or voice shorter and sharper. I would lift my voice and energy would be strong.

This picture shows that a simple move which can help guide students and shows that as a teacher you are fully engaged in the class.

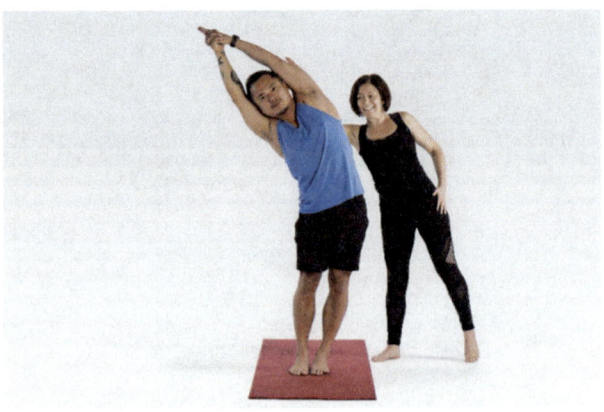

Chapter 7
Demonstration of Poses

Should we demonstrate poses in class?

The question is why would we need to demonstrate a pose? Ideally, we have enough dialogue and our instructions are clear enough that we don't need to show the pose. However, sometimes for the sake of first-time students or if the pose is slightly different to what people normally do, we may need to show the set-up. However, set-up is all we need to show, we don't need to stay in the pose. If you have good dialogue, you should never have an issue talking students through even the most complex of poses. If you decide to demonstrate a pose, you also need to make sure it's in a place where everyone can see you. With 50 people in a hot yoga, this could be impossible so it's preferable to rely on your dialogue as it can reach a lot more people.

How do we teach poses we can't actually do?

There are many reasons why maybe we can't do a pose, i.e., tightness or bone compression or short limbs or maybe we have an injury. That does not mean we can't teach a pose. Why do I say that, well if the issue is I can't show it because

I have short arms that will never change so does that mean I can't ever teach that pose? Of course not. As yoga teachers, we need to know how to do a pose even if we can't actually do it. It's also perfectly okay to tell students you can't do a pose. This is where words are important; if you have the right dialogue, you can teach anything. Of course, there is always an option to use a student to demonstrate but let's assume we don't know all the students then we need to rely on our words so they need to be clear and accurate instructions.

How much of class should we practise with students?

Ideally, as little as possible, you should be able to teach a class without showing anything. There are many reasons why:

- Our job is to teach and help students not show poses.
- If we demonstrate a lot and try to teach, it can be tiring.
- If we are constantly demonstrating postures, we are not able to adjust or take care of our students.

I have been to many classes where the teacher practices the whole class with the students. I completely disagree with this (it's my opinion, maybe yours is different) my job as a teacher, the one I am paid to do is to teach and not practice. My job as a teacher is to help guide students through a yoga class and not use this time for personal practice. I know for some of you this has been the way you have taught for a while, so take the time to improve your dialogue so that you don't need to demonstrate. We need to use our voice and our words, this can get lost if we are actually doing the poses, especially if we have our heads down. Our voices can sound muffled and not clear. If students have their heads down, they also need to hear us clearly so that they don't need to look up. Make the words clear and concise and you don't need to show any pose.

If you do demonstrate ideally, you would only show one side, if you feel the need to demonstrate one side you should not need to do the other. I know what you are thinking will it not make my body imbalanced? Well, as long as you only show the set up it's not enough to have a huge effect. You of course you could choose to demonstrate the weaker or tighter side to help to try to balance your body more, but again this is not the time to focus on you it's time for the students. The reason I say we should just demonstrate one side if we feel the need to is so that we can focus our attention on students and helping them rather than showing how to do it again. Whilst we cue the pose we can go adjust students and help correct their poses. One thing you do need to follow is if you demo a pose is to make sure you do it properly. Quite often we show the set-up of a pose whilst we look at students and we don't think too much about what we are doing. We have to consider that we must show it with the correct alignment according to our body. It does not matter if, for instance, our hips are not square in warrior 2 this might be due to the shape of the pelvis or tight muscles. However, if we show it with a small step and knee going over the ankle it does not set a good example for students. Some students will copy this and then they are set up wrong.

Chapter 8
Room Position

Let's look at room position – Why does this matter? Room position is important for many reasons so let's explore why.

Where is it appropriate to stand?

It's always important to be in a position where you can be seen, i.e., if the students face the left side of the room make sure they can see you. It is not always possible to always be in the position where everyone can see you but where possible it's at least good to be where you can be seen for the setup of the pose. So why does this matter, first-time students find comfort in seeing the teacher. They often don't know what to do and they might not fully understand the instructions so if they can see the teacher then there is a chance the teacher might explain using their body what to do. As a teacher you are able to indicate what you want people to do by using words and even using your own body, i.e., you can show your knee in line with your ankle and point at yourself to help students understand. There will be times you will want to adjust students and you won't be in the position where you can be seen. So my suggestion would be to stand where they can see you for set up and then move to adjust students.

So where is not a good place to stand? It's never good to stand directly behind students who are back-bending, it can be very distracting. Imagine dropping your head back and being faced with a teacher's face. I find a good place to stand when students are back bending is either to the side of the room or at the front. From the side, it's very easy to see people's alignment but at the front, for sure you are not going to distract any students. Another place which is not good to stand is directly in front of students when they are trying to see themselves in the mirror. Sometimes you may need to start here to set up, i.e., if you want to emphasise the grip in a standing bow the front is a good place to stand as many students can see what you are doing. However, once you are set up then move out of the way so they can see in the mirror

See in the picture below as he drops his head back his view is of my groin area so this is not the best place to stand.

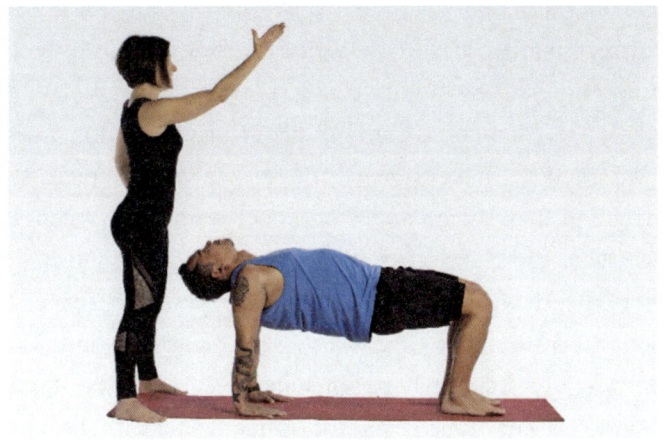

Not only is room position important but how you move around the room is also important.

There are times when you should stand still if possible. When students are balancing, i.e., standing on one leg, we should stand still as much as possible because teachers moving around can be very distracting when trying to balance. Find a place where you can stand still without being a distraction. If you do need to move, then do it without creating haste so do not rush unless you have to and not too close to students' mats where possible.

Understand personal space

We should try to avoid standing on students' mats as much as possible. It is possible to adjust someone without standing on a mat. Sometimes it can't be helped but do try to avoid it if you can. Their mat is their personal space and by standing on their mat we invade that space. I know as a teacher I don't really want to stand on somcone's sweaty mat. I have taught in many studios where, after I walk out my feet are dirty, I don't necessarily want a teacher with dirty feet to stand on my mat, especially if it's my own personal mat.

As yoga teachers, we do get physically close to students but we need to make sure we do it in a professional way. Understand their space and your space and know when you adjust what parts of your body are coming into contact with their body. If we enter into someone's personal space, we need to ensure it's for the right reasons and done professionally. Stand where you can safely adjust the student without invading their space too much. Ensure that you are not standing with parts of your body in their face, in particular, your sexual parts i.e., Groin, buttocks or a female chest.

How to move around the room

Most of the time whilst teaching, we will be moving around the room. There are many ways to do this, I know what you're thinking we have to think about how we move around? Having a teacher pace up and down can be distracting, or one that circles around the room constantly can make students feel unbalanced. You want to make sure you have a reason to move around the room and of course, it's important to share energy so you do want to move around the room. A good suggestion would be to work the corners, i.e., spend some time on the right side and then change to the left. Which we would naturally do when people face different directions anyway. Most of the time during teaching, I would be towards the back so as to ensure that I am not in the way and they can use the mirror to see their own pose. The mirror is a useful tool to help students correct their poses. I have also taught at studios where there is no mirror. In situations like this, I would be stationed more towards the front of the room so I can help guide students. You also don't want to stand in one spot for a long time but move around when it's appropriate. Of course, some of these suggestions are also irrelevant if you need to attend to a student, so if you think a student looks like they might faint or is feeling unwell and everyone is in a balancing pose of course you should attend to that student. These suggestions are for when all is good in a class and these are ideas to improve how we deliver a class.

Chapter 9
Adjustments

Should we offer adjustments in class?

This can be a tricky subject according to where in the world you live. I have taught in the west and also in Asia and for sure in Asia; they are much more open to adjustments. In fact, here they expect it and really appreciate being adjusted.

The first thing you should always do is ask permission. Child's pose is a great opportunity to find out who is or isn't comfortable with tactile adjustments. Ideally, you have asked before class but if you did not; I find it so much more comfortable to ask students when they are not looking. That way it takes the pressure off someone if they don't want to be adjusted so they don't need to feel embarrassed by saying no. Some studios have discs that you place next to your mat, which say whether the teacher can adjust you, or not. This is also a nice idea.

How to adjust students

There are two types of adjustments:

1. Corrective – correcting a student's alignment, are their feet in the wrong place.
2. Deeper – These adjustments are to help students who can't go any further by themselves and need help.

So assuming you have permission you are now able to help adjust students. Even though some students will say yes be aware, they can change their minds and that's okay.

One thing to consider is you don't want to startle a student, by turning up next to them and then suddenly you have hands on them. What I do is when I approach the student I make my breathing louder so they are aware of my presence, especially if they can't see me i.e., in a downward dog. I might also initially move to where they can see me i.e., walk around the back of them in a downward dog and then move around to the front. I might also place a foot or hand where they can see it so they are aware that I intend to help them. Once I commit to putting my hands on a student I do it with a firm touch. Sometimes students will relax when you place your hands on them so make sure it's a firm touch so that you can support them if you need it.

It's important to also read resistance; you can feel it energetically when you go near someone. If you get the feeling, they don't want to be touched just walk away, or even if they say no. Don't take it personally some people prefer not to be touched. We also don't know what happened that day and each day is different they might just need space that day and that's fine.

Ask for feedback, I will often lower my voice so I speak directly to the student and maybe say, "Does your back feel okay? Can I push a little more?" You will know when you can, there will be resistance and you might find they just hold their breath so remind them to breathe. I might also say, "Does it feel okay?" Which most of the time it does but I ask as much as possible to give them the chance to change their mind if it's too strong or too deep. I would rather someone say no and I easy off than they end up hurt. Generally, I never go too far and I always make sure that if I am helping to stretch their hamstrings, I can actually feel their hamstrings so I can feel when it's pulling too much.

If you decide to adjust someone, make sure you are confident, don't do it half-heartedly or lightly, make sure you know what to do and do it with confidence. Students will know if you are unsure and then they will have doubts. So be sure if you do adjust you know exactly where to stand and what to do. If you are not confident, just teach and focus on your words and don't adjust until you know you are comfortable.

Unless you are giving specific instructions to that individual, it's good to say what you are doing, for instance, if you help someone in child's pose by pushing their hips down, say what you are doing. This way you can verbally correct many students at the same time, this also helps the student you are adjusting to understand what you are doing to them.

"Lengthen the hips to heels."

"Stretch the back by reaching the arms away from the hips."

Know your students

Before you even go near someone to adjust them, you need to know their bodies. I have a rule that I don't touch anyone in their first class with me unless they are about to hurt their selves. To give good adjustments, you need to know the following: the student's strength, flexibility, body type and any injuries.

Sometimes the adjustments require you to stand quite close to the student and require may require you to put your hands on the student. You need to be sure that this is done in a professional way.

Picture 1 is not the best place to stand, my face is pointed directly at his groin. Pic 2 is much better, I can adjust his hips in a more professional way. Below you will also see that when I am being adjusted in warrior 2, the teacher's face is directly in front of my pelvis. It's better to adjust from behind like in picture 2.

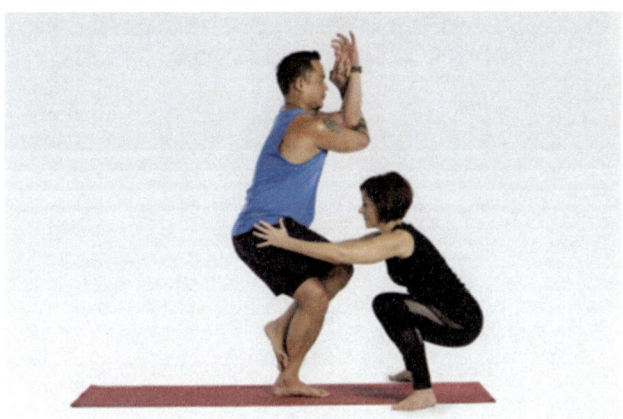

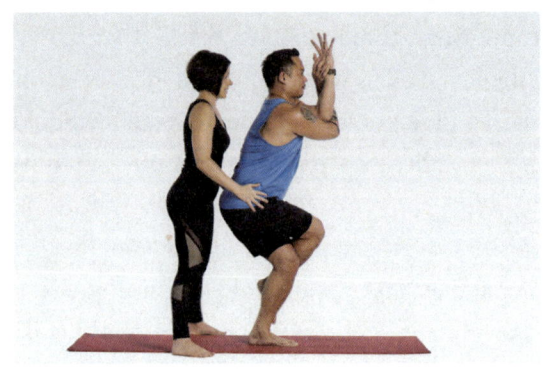

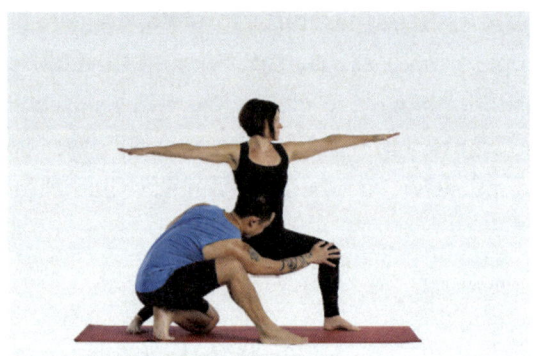

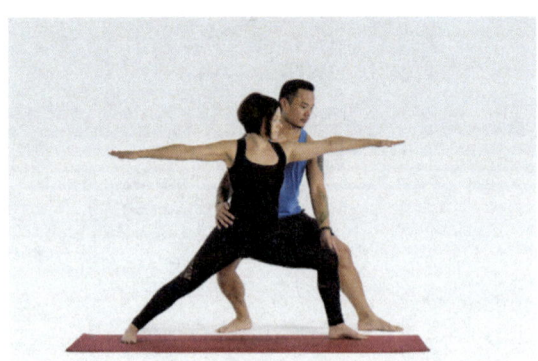

Adjustments

You will also see from the picture below that the teacher's hands are very close to my chest you have to be very careful when placing your hands here it's easy to slip. It would be better to have the hand lower on the ribcage. The other picture is just wrong, he is pulling my hand, which is not good for the shoulder joint, and his foot is on top of mine, which is a little impolite.

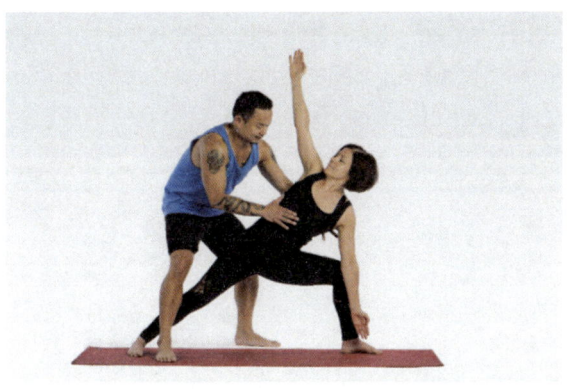

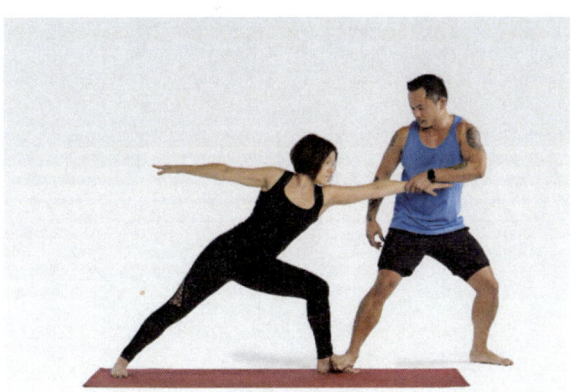

Adjustments

In picture 1 below, you can see that I have my hand on his lower back, which I want to lengthen the other hand is on the shoulder to assist in lengthening the spine. I could have put my knee down so I don't need to lean forward however I am not very tall and I would not generate the same power if I am below him that I would if I was above him. In picture 2, you can see I have placed one knee down so you can see that I am also considering how I stand to ensure I am not going to hurt myself either. My top hand helps him to feel what I want him to stretch whilst the opposite hand prevents him from sinking so he gets to feel the stretch.

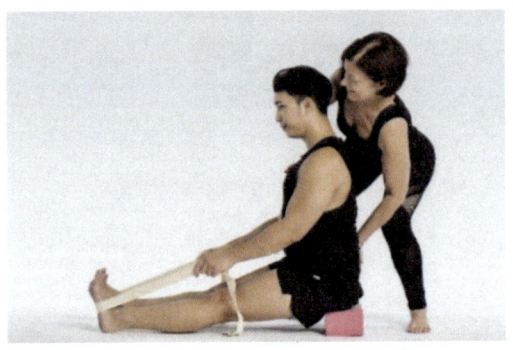

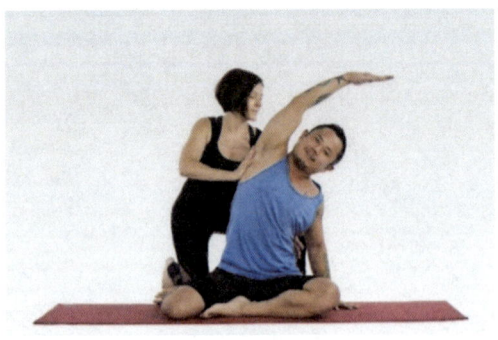

Adjustments

Know the strength of the student and meet that strength. If I am adjusting a big strong guy, I need to know that I am able to help assist him without injuring myself. I also need to know that I have the strength to help get him to go further or deeper. At the same time, you may adjust someone who is not as strong as you so you need to not push as hard. Make sure your adjustment is firm, the touch should be firm and not light. You are not stroking a cat but at the same time you are not trying to stuff the bin with more rubbish so just know what level of pressure you need to use.

Know the limitations of the student; it's important to know how far you can help them, without pushing too far. Feedback from the student always helps with this. It's important to move students into deeper places with awareness. What joint are you moving how does this affect other joints' muscles etc. Someone may have flexibility in one direction but that does not mean that have it in all directions.

Every person has a different body type hence we do not look the same in the same pose. If we have an understanding of body types, then it makes it easier to understand why some things are harder. Someone with long arms finds it easier to bind than someone with short arms. There are so many factors, limb length, body length, muscle tightness, bone structure and so much more that affect how we move into poses. If we have a better understanding, then we can help students understand more about their own practice.

Injuries

This is one of the most important subject areas but also the most complicated. Sometimes people come to yoga for the first time after they have been injured, maybe because the doctor told them to go to yoga or because they want to move and they realise they can't do something more strenuous. Of course, there are also regular students who simply incur an injury and they don't want to stop practising yoga.

The one thing I have learned over the years of teaching, people seem to associate yoga teachers with doctors. They turn up with scans from a doctor or a letter from their physiotherapist, which states that they have torn their anterior cruciate ligament or they have an L4 disk herniation. This is the very reason I feel that yoga teachers need to be better equipped with anatomy knowledge. The question is do you know what to do with these two issues? Or do you know what further questions to ask? The first thing that I would say is, to be honest, and if you don't know how to deal with them please tell your students. The one question you should ask is, "Did your doctor clear you for yoga?"

If yes, then accept them and explain that they should modify, as they need to be. You should also ask if a student has taken painkillers. If they have you probably don't want them in class, painkillers prevent someone from feeling pain therefore, they could go too far and potentially make the injury worse.

On a simple level, you could ask how does this movement feel? Or did the doctor give you any exercises for rehab? I.e., for the disk herniation depending on which direction the disc has moved spinal extension could be good or could be bad. The safest way is to keep the spine in a neutral position. The best option is to ensure you have a good knowledge of anatomy and don't try to diagnose something when you don't understand it. We are not doctors but having a basic understanding of how to deal with injuries is key then at least we know how to modify the pose. I will also refrain from any adjustments with someone with an injury just letting them move at the pace they need to. This is an extremely big and complicated topic and is possibly a book in itself.

My general rule is when a student first comes to my class, I don't do any adjustments to them. I don't know anything about their body so I am not in a place to help move them deeper until I have an understanding of their body. It's important to also not make the new student feel intimidated i.e., you are doing it all wrong so I will correct you on every pose. Let them move and acknowledge them so you have made them feel welcome but let them see how it feels at first. One thing we need to remember as a teacher is that we have a group class, sometimes we can get very fixated on fixing a specific student, i.e., they are in warrior 2 and we adjust every single part of their body during which time everyone else is waiting. We have to always remember to, as much as we can, give equal attention to all students as possible. Of course, you won't have time or need to adjust every student but just make sure it's not always the same one all the time.

Chapter 10
Class Structure

Basic class structure

If you attend a teacher-training course that has a set sequence, which is common in hot yoga style training, then at first, you don't need to think too much about sequencing as you will teach what you have learned on the course at first. However, after a while, you might decide to venture into other styles and there might be a need to teach classes which don't have a set sequence. If you have attended a hot-style teacher training which includes more static postures, i.e., holding for a period of time, then you might not have been taught how to construct a flow-style class. So where do you begin, you may need to learn other postures and different styles but keep it simple, to begin with.

I would always start with a basic warm-up like the one below.

- Child pose
- Cat cow
- Shoulder rotation
- Downward dog

- Ragdoll

It does not need to be exactly like this and does not need to take very long. I find this is a good way to start for a couple of reasons:

- It tells me a lot about people's bodies and what they are capable of. Is their spine tight or do they have shoulders tight, how is their hamstring length?
- Child's pose is a good start just to centre yourself especially if you rushed from work. It's also a good chance to ask about adjustments without anyone having to be embarrassed to say no.
- Finally, if someone comes into class late they have not missed a major part of the class just the simple warm-up. Each studio has its own policy on lateness some allow it and some don't.

Sun salutations:

- Learn how to teach sun salutations. Although you don't need to include them in all flow classes, they are a great addition to flow classes. Sun salutations are a great way to mobilise and warm the whole body. If you ever get stuck in a class or you forget your sequence, a sun salutation will give you some breathing space. They are also great ways to transition from pose to pose if you want to teach a more dynamic class. There are many types of sun salutations, start with the basic sun salutation A and then explore other options.

After this, you want to follow a basic structure of standing poses, seated poses, prone poses and then finally supine poses. It does not need to be exactly like this but you don't want to have people supine and then suddenly have to come to a stand; it does not always make sense. Once you get down to a supine position, then energy will change and it's hard to lift it again if students are tired.

So how to structure a class in terms of which poses to do, there are many factors to consider:

- Is the group beginners or more intermediate?
- What time of day is the class taking place?
- How long is the class?
- Will I have a mixed-level group?
- Does the class have a name?

So that are some actual factors to consider which we will examine but then you need to consider what you want to achieve from the class, i.e., relaxing and stretching or strength and power. It's very important to know your audience, you might have a group of triathletes one day and over 60s the next day. I know what you're thinking: the triathletes need the power class and the over 60s need the stretch, but that's not always the case. If those over the 60s have done yoga for many years, they can be pretty strong and flexible, whereas the triathletes might be strong but they could be super tight. We should never make an assumption based on someone's age or body type. See them move then decide. I can remember teaching side plank in class once, the 60-year-old lady held it without moving, it was no issue for her, the 25-year-old guy with a ripped body was shaking like a leaf, you just can't assume.

The most important thing to consider when planning a class is to have a backup plan as you may need to digress or progress according to who turns up for class. So you need to know modifications to make it easier or more challenging.

Mistakes often made by new teachers

- We need to teach 'advanced' poses.
- We need to show that we can be super creative.
- We need to show off how well we can do advanced poses.
- We need to make our classes super tough.
- We need to be spiritual.

The ability to teach 'advanced' poses in class depends on the group but most of the time majority of the class can't actually do the 'advanced' poses. In order to teach 'advanced' poses, you need to know what you must prepare before doing the pose i.e., which parts of the body need to be open or warmed up. You also need to know how to help students who can't do it. Furthermore, what is advanced, most think it's some fancy arm balance, or where we wrap our legs behind our head. Depending on your body structure even simple poses can feel like they are advanced for some people. Focus on the essence of yoga mindful movement and hold poses longer to make people work harder. Understand that if one person in class can achieve it and the others can't then there is no point in teaching it.

Showing that we can be super creative is nice but more often than not, students actually like to practice regular poses. This is why set sequences are popular. It's great to be creative but there should be a purpose to it, other than just being fancy i.e., the pose order makes sense and the flow works. I feel I get a much better response when I teach them something and get them to understand where to feel it and get them to understand what is the purpose.

Showing off, how well we can do advanced poses is something that lots of teachers feel they need to do. Just showing a simple warrior 2 never seems enough especially with social media. But why does it matter what we can do? There might be many reasons why a teacher can't do a pose but that does not mean they cannot teach that pose. Teaching yoga is about knowing your limitations, understanding your and students' bodies and taking them safely through practice. It's not about showing off and dropping into splits. We often feel the need to show something in order to validate why we are a teacher, but if we can safely guide students through a class what does it matter what we can and cannot do as long as we practice what we preach.

One lesson I learned whilst teaching is with regards to making our classes tough. I knew I could not do all the fancy poses but I felt I needed to show something so I made my classes tough. For some, this was okay they loved it but for others, it did not work. I got away with it because I was super nice always. For sure, some students did not come back to my class because it was too hard. Some of the best teachers teach simple things and are successful. I knew that because I could not teach fancy stuff at that time, I could make people feel it by holding simple poses for a long time i.e., warrior 2. If you consider the reasons why people come to class, they want to destress, they want to get strong, or maybe they want to stretch. Find your balance in your class. If you go too far in one direction, it can lose students' interest. Even for me if I go to class and it's too 'easy' for me, I might not go back.

Of course, there is the argument that if too easy is too difficult for me then it's what I need. This is true but it won't necessarily keep me interested. It's a hard balance to find, but I often find people will teach the style they prefer to practice, so my classes are not easy as such but I know how to balance and change them according to the group in the room.

Teach the class in the room it's a simple point but important. You might have planned a super advanced class but if Auntie May and her buddies turn up for a class it might not be the right class to teach and you need to change it immediately. So, you should always be prepared because even though the schedule says vinyasa flow, it might be the only time Auntie May and her buddies are able to come to class so you need to adapt. Of course, you don't change the class just for one person but make sure you have options and modifications if there is that one person or a small group of people in the class.

If the class is mixed level, who do you cater for? This is always a tricky point do you cater for the two new people or the 12 advanced students. Of course, the reverse can also happen. The general rule is to cater for the majority, but it's very simple if have modifications and options then this will not be an issue. You need to make the new and old students feel welcome and they need to have a good experience. I always take the idea if I am teaching something challenging and most of the class can't do it, the class level is wrong and

I need to change it. If there are two people sitting on their mat watching, it's okay but if 12 people are watching the three people that can do it, my class is wrong. This is where you need to see the level and adjust accordingly and not just teach what you planned.

So how do you know the right level? The start of class tells you a lot, about how flexible they are and what they can do. If you observe, you can see very easily what the group can do, for instance, if most of the class can't hold plank this gives you a good idea of what students can do. You can probably safely say that a forearm balance is out of the question. However, at the other end of the scale, if everyone is jumping back and achieving chaturanga easily then maybe a stretch-style class might not be what they want. I find a simple warm-up and sun salutations are a good indication of what people can do. You can see easily if they are strong and how flexible they are in certain areas. Bear in mind a hamstring stretch for someone who is tight, can feel just as hard as a plank does for someone who is not so strong.

Teach what students need, we tend to like doing the things that are easy; they make us look and feel good. In reality, we need a balance of what we need and what we want. For me, flexion of the mid-thoracic and lumbar spine is super hard, and in reality, I don't want to do rabbit pose because it's so hard but it's exactly what my body needs. I can hold a plank or do a push-up with ease but it's not what my body needs and therefore does not challenge me in the same way. Therein lies the tricky part of teaching, giving people what they need but also giving them the feel-good factor of what they want. By watching people during a simple warm-up or sun salutations, you can see if they are tight in their shoulders, they lack spinal mobility, or they have tight hips or hamstrings. Now, of course, as a new teacher just teaching is hard enough, don't even imagine to try to look for these things and adjust your class but if you have been teaching for a while it's easy to see these things and you can adjust a few things accordingly.

I also find it useful to take into account where we are during the year. Reality is near the holiday season people socialise more and possibly do less yoga. Lots of eating and sitting watching TV means hips and hamstrings get tighter. In January, my classes might focus on more core, and maybe more stretching, from all the sitting that has been done and chances are people did not work out so much. Whereas in the summer, people are more active and can cope with a more dynamic class.

In order to be recognised as a real yogi, we must be spiritual and we should chant, play yogic music and always use Sanskrit names. This is by no means a criticism of anyone who does these things, but let's come back to being the true representation of you. If it's not your character to talk about the light within you and chant, then don't do it. Not every yoga class needs to include chakra cleansing. The reality is for most it's a movement class that makes people feel good. I learned myself coming from teaching in the west to the east my teaching changed so much. In the UK, we did long meditations, chakra cleansing and all that fun stuff. Once I got to Bangkok yoga was more fitness based. The local culture meant that people went to the temple and they had their spiritual moments so there was no need to address it in class. Whereas in the UK everyone was stressed and they no longer went to church so it was welcomed. The whole idea of meditation after or during class was so important in the UK yet in Bangkok people did this themselves so there was no need. You have to also think about the group you are teaching, the over 60s might not be so stressed out so don't feel the need to meditate so much, the new generation spends so much time on social media looking at what they want to be and stressed about how they look and feel that maybe positive mediation is very useful.

How to structure a class?

This is much easier if you have students who are new to yoga. Because warrior 2 is a new pose to them so it's something they might get excited about, whereas the seasoned yogi might be less excited. You have a chance to construct a bunch of flows that include standard poses and the new students won't get bored. You can do all the variations of warrior flows and people will be happy. The reality is normally class is a mixed group of individuals which include new, experienced and anywhere in between.

We always feel that students want to see something different from us each time. But if you look at the numbers of people that follow the Ashtanga primary series or a hot series they do the same thing every day. There is some comfort in that, we know what to do, we know what to expect and we can see our progression in each part of the class. Of course, there are some who prefer to do different style classes each time. If you teach at the same studio each week or maybe you just teach at one studio multiple times a week, students will start to expect to see a different style of class. Unless the schedule indicates it's a set sequence then students will expect to see different things.

There are a few ways to design a class:

1. A themed class, i.e., twisting or hip opener.
2. Reverse engineering.
3. Simple basic class.

No 1 is pretty straight forward i.e., you come up with an idea for a class and then you structure your class around that theme, taking into account the order in which makes sense for poses to be taught. I would make sure that I include the theme throughout the class. So if I were to design a twisting class although this is not a full-length class it gives you the idea of how you can theme a class:

Child's pose.
Cat cow five rounds.
Shoulder rotations/twist.
Downward dog. (Can add a twist, grab the opposite ankle)
Sun salutation A.
Sun Salutation B – with high lunge variation.
Round 1 – Regular lunge and add prayer twist.
Round 2 – Twisted lunge with arms wide into prayer twist.
Round 3 – Lunge twist and back bend into a reverse warrior.
Round 4 – High lunge twist into a twisted half-moon.
Separate leg stretch – twist.
Twisted goddess pose.
Twisted triangle.
Standing big toe pose with twist.
Vinyasa to the mat.
Seated forward fold with twist.

Sage pose twist.
Boat with twist.
Pigeon twist.
Supine twist.

Justin Flow sequence

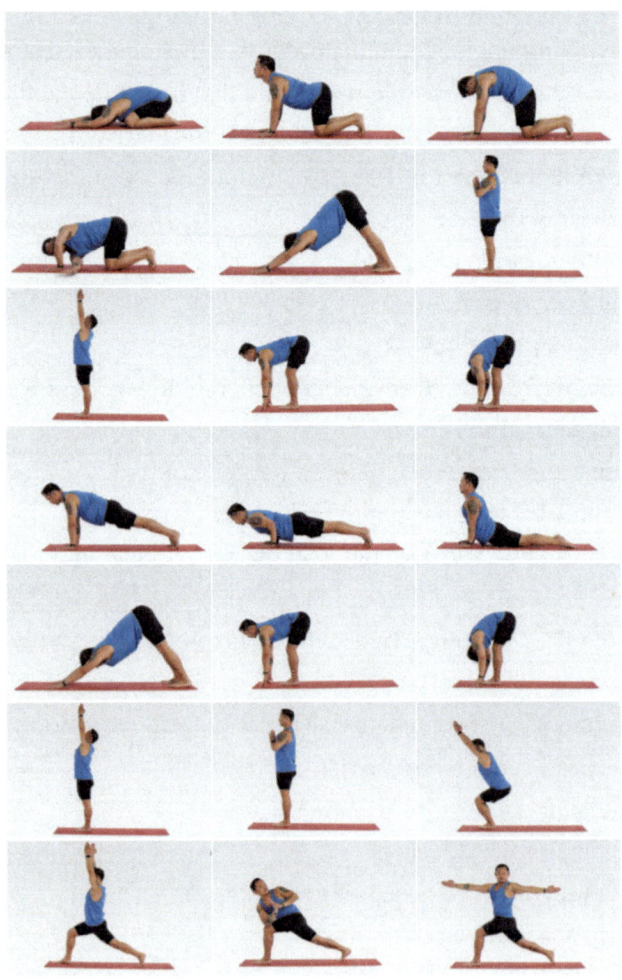

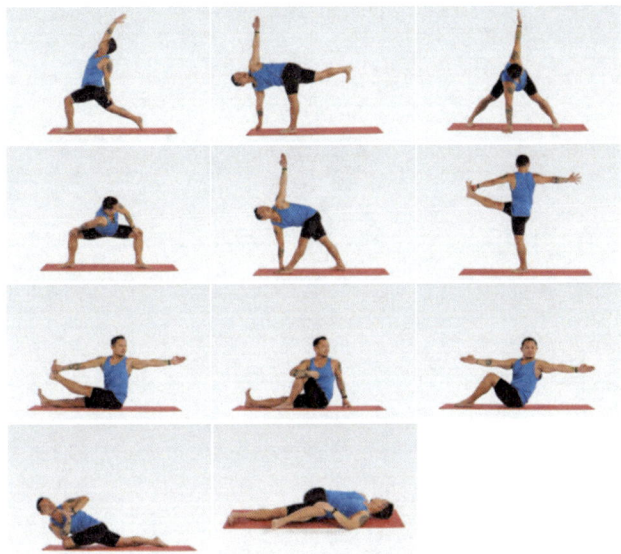

Reverse engineering – Bird of paradise

In some ways, I find this an easier way to design a class. This is when you find your peak pose, which is normally something challenging and you design the class around that pose. So, you need to think about what parts of the body mobilised and strengthened in order to achieve this pose. Let's look at what is happening in the bird of paradise pose.

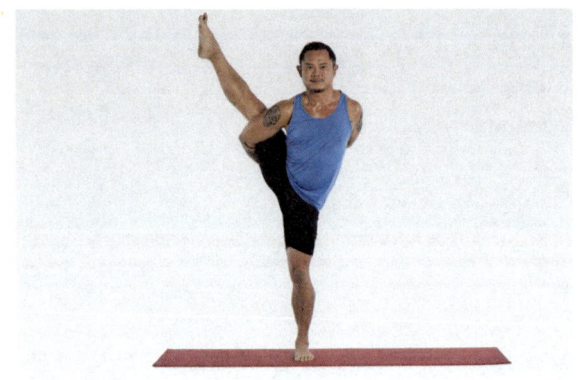

Yoga

So what do we need to mobilise or open?

- Ankles
- Hips
- Shoulders
- Hamstrings
- Spine

Lifted leg – Muscles that are stretching:

- Hamstrings
- Adductors
- Gluteus

Lifted leg – Muscles that are contracting:
- Quadriceps
- Hip flexors

- External rotators

Front Arm – Muscles that are contracting:

- Biceps
- Internal rotators

Opposite arm – Muscles that are lengthening:

- Deltoids
- Biceps
- Serratus anterior
- Pec Major
- Upper traps

Muscles that need to be contracted to stabilise the body:

- Obliques on the opposite side to the lifted leg.
- Rectus abdominus on the opposite side to the lifted leg.
- Quadratus lumborum on the opposite side to the lifted leg.
- Calf muscles of the standing leg.
- Adductors of the standing leg.
- Quadriceps of the standing leg.
- Gluteus of the standing leg.

So in order to achieve the pose, a number of joints need to be mobilised, and muscles need to be stretched and strengthened. So it's very simple how to prepare your class you need to open hips, shoulders and hamstrings. So poses like eagle, butterfly, cow face, low lunge, seated forward fold, standing big toe pose and many more. Spend the first ¾ of class preparing the body bird of paradise then finish with a nice cool down and relaxation.

Factors to consider when structuring a class

The way I structure my simple class is easy, I start with a warm, up i.e., moving the spine in all directions, flexion, extension, lateral flexion and rotation. Almost everyone needs spinal mobility. I start with standing poses, seated poses, prone poses and finally supine. I might choose a simple theme like shoulder opening and will spend the class focused on that. Like above, I will always have a peak pose, it does not always need to be very challenging just a point in which I need to prepare the body prior to doing it in order to achieve the best results.

So if I decide that bird of paradise is my pose of choice and I see very early on that everyone has super tight hips or hamstrings then I might need to adjust my class, because if no one can even get close to a bird of paradise it's a waste of time teaching it. If you get to the point in class where two people are doing the pose and 10 are sitting on their mats watching you have lost the majority of the group and it does not make for a good class experience. So maybe your peak pose is simply a triangle with a bind or move into some deeper hip opener poses.

I find by following this structure, makes it easier to decide what poses should come before this. The peak pose is always about ¾ of the way through the class in order to get to the peak with then enough time to slow and cool down towards the end. Sometimes the peak pose might be even something as simple as a forearm plank. It does not need to be fancy it just needs to be the pose you have chosen as a peak pose or focus of class for today.

So other factors to consider when planning a class is:

- How long is the warm-up /cool-down?
- Do we include mediation and if so, how long should that be?
- Do we chant ohm?
- What about Namaste?
- Should I play music?
- What about breathing exercises?

How long is the warm-up and cool-down?

It really depends on how long the actual class is, the shorter the class the quicker they are. As a general rule, the warm-up and cool-down should be around five minutes for each part and may be extended to 10 for longer classes. See the section below about class length.

Do we include meditation?

Sometimes factors like this can be determined based on where in the world you live. The reason I say this is because teaching in the west was very different to teaching in the east for me. When I taught in the UK, students liked the idea of meditation and in fact, in most of my 90-minute classes, 15–25 minutes was meditation at the end of class. Once I moved to Bangkok, this would not be suitable for the clients here.

The culture here is people go to the temple to pray or meditate so when it came to yoga they wanted to focus on the more physical aspect. So even though they actually took to mediation much easier the mediation part was never as long. You also need to consider if you are comfortable teaching meditation. This is important because if you are not comfortable teaching it then don't include it. It's not a requirement of class to include it, I would say it's much better to teach from the heart and be genuine. Meditation does not also need to be a long drawn-out story or visualisation it can be simply sitting in silence focusing on the breath. Later in the book, I will include some sample meditations you can use. Mediation can be done at the start of class or at the end of class. Initially, the physical aspect of yoga came about because the focus was meditation and stillness. In order to sit in a comfortable position for long periods of time, it required the hips to be very open. In India where people were used to sitting in this tailor-crossed position, their hips were naturally more open. As more western people came to yoga, it became more apparent that more mobility would be required on the hips. Hence, the physical aspect came first and meditation came after class.

- Do we chant ohm?
- What about Namaste?

Again, these two are very personal and if you don't feel comfortable doing it then you don't need to do it. You can always come up with your own version of something special if you feel like you would like to at the end of class. I don't always chant ohm and I know many teachers who do and many who don't. Not all teachers finish with Namaste either they often have their own version of special messages things like "the light in me honours the light in you." I would often say things like "thank yourself for your practice today and thank you for sharing your practice with me." Remember to be yourself and honour your beliefs and don't try to be something you are not.

- Should I play music?

I would say this depends on the style of class you are teaching. If you are teaching a dialogue-based class like hot, I would say it's best not to as it can be a distraction. For other style classes, it's very much a personal choice. Sometimes it's a good distraction from the odd moments of silence but if it's going to distract you or take your attention then maybe don't use it. Sometimes it's nice to include it at the end when it's final relaxation time. Of course, there is always the issue of where you teach and do you need a public performance license. In the UK, I needed to have a PPL license and even with that, I should play royalty-free music. Music is a personal choice and there are no rules so do what feels good. If you play music does it need to be, 'bong bang bong' music i.e., spiritual yoga music, not necessarily like I say just be true to who you are always and you will find the right balance.

- What about breathing exercises?

These are a great addition to class and they don't need to be complicated to teach. Sometimes having people just pause and focus on their own breathing can bring so many benefits.

I will include some simple breathing techniques later in the book. They can be done at the start or the end of class, there are no rules.

I find it so much easier to plan and prepare classes if you have a theme, of course, you don't need to announce it to students but have it in mind, i.e., shoulder opener, hip opener, twisting, detox or stretch and destress. If I set a theme, then it's easier to design a class. So you might say this week we are working on twisting and all your classes include a twisting element. Not only does it make your life easier as a teacher it also shows you have prepared a class rather than just turn up and wing it. Which for someone who has been teaching for many years is easy to do, but I do find preparing makes my life so much easier. I document all my classes for many reasons, one it gives me the chance to look back and use again further in the future if I need to. It is also so I can check what I did last week so I don't repeat the same thing each time. Students like it if you turn up with a theme; it shows you have taken time to think about what to teach. So the question is can you take a cheat sheet into class, why not I say. Of course, if you can memorise your sequence, it's better, but if it's changing, that's not always possible, but showing that you have planned your class is never a bad thing.

Two important aspects about what level of class you teach are what time of day the class is and how long. This is very important, as classes at different times of the day will attract different clientele and you need to prepare based on that. The 7 am class might attract working people who have very little time to work out but they come to practise early every morning. The 9 am class is likely to be the mums who just dropped the kids off at school. The 2 pm class could be students or even the retired generation. Each of those classes should reflect the clients. It's not just the clients that might come it's also how people are feeling at certain times of the day. For me in Bangkok, the 7 am crew were super serious and strong; they came every day and were dedicated. In the UK, the evening classes were more popular and the strong crowd came at night.

Class length can vary from 45 minutes to 60 minutes to 90 minutes. So how different should it be, well, if you have 90 minutes, you can take your time and start reasonably slow and build on the class as time goes on. If you only have 45 minutes, you can't really spend 10–15 minutes slowly warming everyone up, as that's $1/3^{rd}$ of the class gone already. If that's the only class students are going to do that day, then make it worthwhile for them and get them moving quickly. A short five minutes warm if sufficient. If you just do a five minutes warm-up in a 90 minutes class, you might find after 60 minutes people are tired so it's much better to pace the class a bit more. You have to also consider if you plan to do meditation or a breathing exercise at the end and how long will you spend on that. When planning class, it's always best to over plan i.e., have too much prepared and then cut off where needed. When you first start teaching, we are often nervous and what tends to happen is we teach too fast, so always better to have too much so you don't panic about what to do next, you have a backup plan.

Does the time-of-day matter? For me yes, it does. In the morning, we have not moved much we are likely to be stiffer so you don't want to rush into strong dynamic movement or deep stretching without some warm-up. Whereas later in the day, we have at least moved around during the day so the body is a bit more open. Classes later in the day i.e., 6 pm tend to be a bit more dynamic than they would be at 7 am. For classes that are later in the evening i.e., 8 pm, I might start a little more dynamic but I would slow down for the second half so that people don't leave the studio hyped up as it's getting nearer to the time they would sleep, so I might encourage a more relaxed practice to slow down. A lunchtime class would be much like an evening class people are more awake and I possibly would not spend as much time on relaxation, as people need to go back to work after. So you don't want to make the too chilled out. Of course, there are no set rules for any of this it's just something I tend to follow as a rough guide. You have to look at the audience too and who comes to each class. I found in Bangkok the 7am crew were strong strong and although I might start a little slower I would push them as they only have 45 minutes and they want to leave feeling good.

Does the class name make difference? If the class is listed as gentle flow class then of course you should not teach power vinyasa. However, you should also teach the group that is in the room but bear in mind the class name. If everyone in the class is super strong, should you then change it to a stronger class, not necessarily as students might just feel like doing gentle flow. It is also possible that this is the only time they could come and they did not check the name they just came. This is where your instinct comes in and you have to get a feel for the class that does not mean that you start teaching a vinyasa flow class. Your instinct will tell you but maybe keep it simple, but do some deep long stretches so students walk out feeling good although they might not have done 20 chaturangas, their hips feel super open or their back and so consequently they feel like they did something good. Get feedback from students too i.e., do you want it harder next time or more gentle. If it's your own, class what name do you give it? We always think we need to come up with some fancy name for a yoga class but most of the time simple ones work, i.e., vinyasa or Hatha or gentle flow. If I go to a studio I don't know and I see vinyasa, I have a good idea what level it might be.

Does the day of the week matter?

Ideally no but much like the time, I do take this into account, on a Monday morning, people might be more tired and their bodies might be tighter than let's say a Thursday evening. In a Sunday afternoon class, you might want to slow things down a little as people get ready for a new week ahead. Friday evening is after a week at work and so again although not the same as Sunday I might be more inclined to relax a little more. Saturday morning, I find there tend to be two types of people who come to class, those that want to start their weekend well and have a busy day ahead and those that maybe had a late Friday night and are feeling a little delicate. I don't honestly change my classes a huge amount other than Monday classes and maybe Sunday afternoon but these are things to think about when you plan your classes. Power vinyasa might not be the ideal class for a 7 am Monday morning class. It also might not be the right class for a Sunday afternoon, I find a popular style class on Sunday afternoon is Yin yoga.

How about different times of the year or seasons?

The time of the year can also be a factor to consider. December is considered party month and often people do less yoga and maybe indulge a little more and so by the time January comes people might not have done as much yoga. I also find that people are keen to lose the weight they gained over the holiday period. So for either option the first week back might be challenging so I tend to start a little slower and build people up towards the later part of the month.

Seasons

Of course, this is only applicable in countries where there are clear seasons, i.e., spring summer, autumn and winter. I have found during winter people tend to slow down a little whereas in the summer there tends to be more energy. So my focus for winter classes especially in the run-up to the holiday season tends to slow a little as people tend to be stressed about running around getting things done. In the summer, the evenings are lighter and people tend to venture out more and I find people have more energy maybe from extra sunlight.

I know what you are thinking, now I need to think about the time of the class, the people in the class, the day of the week and the time of the year. It's all too much. As a new teacher, you don't need to think about any of these but these are just some ideas that you can consider implementing once you get more confident in teaching.

Chapter 11
Breathing Exercises/Pranayama

Pranayama or breathing exercises are a great addition to the class. Anything extra along with the actual physical practice is always a great thing to add to class but you need to be confident that you know what you're doing. So I will always say keep it simple and only teach things you feel fully confident in. It might mean that you start with the simple things like inhaling for x count, then hold and exhale for x count. However, there are many versions you can learn and teach once you are more confident.

Benefits of breathing exercises

There are so many benefits to pranayama:

- Helps to connect body and mind.
- Increased lung function.
- Improves cardiovascular health.
- Strengthen the immune system.
- Improves mental concentration.

Breathing is so important for many factors in life, of course, the obvious factor is that it keeps us alive. Breathing is an instinctive action we do not need to control it in any way, however, it is also voluntary in that we can control how we breathe to a certain extent. There are three types of breathing we tend to use high mid and low breathing.

High breathing – is focused on breathing into the upper chest around the clavicle area. This is one of the most common forms of breathing for adults today. This focuses on the top $1/3^{rd}$ of the lungs only. Women who are pregnant and people with big tummies will tend to breathe like this.

Mid-breathing – is focused on breathing into the thoracic area, expanding the ribcage laterally and this tends to focus on the mid-part of the lungs. Opening and stretching the intercostal muscles will make this type of breathing easier.

Low breathing – More commonly called diaphragmatic or belly breathing, focuses on breathing into the low part of the lungs. The belly will rise and fall with each inhale and exhale.

These forms of breathing use only part of the lungs and respiratory system. The complete Yoga breath uses all of these forms; it ensures that every part of the lung and the respiratory muscles are used within a breath.

During the complete full yoga breath, on the inhalation the diaphragm contracts which generates a little pressure on our internal organs, this pressure is in effect a gentle massage on the organs and helps them to function correctly. As we exhale, the diaphragm relaxes and the ribs drawback in and down. Hence, it's good to stretch the muscles around the ribs so that they can expand and relax to full capacity.

Most people only use about 1/10th of their lung capacity, which is adequate to exist but not enough to ensure high vitality levels and well-being. So including breathing can help students increase the capacity of their lungs.

Our breath rhythm changes during exercise, often it can become shallower and faster. Our breathing tends to alter to high chest breathing when exercising. Which is why our breath is faster than our regular breath. When we breathe in this way, less air goes into our lungs. When we breathe fast like this, it can also increase our heart rate, which can trigger our sympathetic nervous system to come into action. Which is the opposite of what we want to achieve in yoga, we want to slow the heart and the breath. What is clever about some yoga poses is that they can increase the heart rate without changing the breath. So the heart gets stronger without the body being completely fatigued.

- On average, we inhale/exhale 16 times per minute whilst at rest, during this time ½ litre of air is taken in and exhaled.
- With the correct full breathing, we are able to increase this to 3 ½ litres of air inhaled and exhaled.

½ Litre V 3.5 Litres

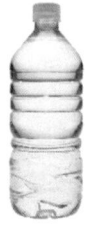
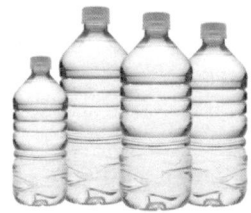

Most of the time we don't breathe as deep as we can, therefore not using the full lung capacity.

- So what are the benefits of deep breathing?
- How do you use the full lung capacity?
- What can restrict us?
- What types of breathing should we do in yoga?
- Breathing and the nervous system.

So what are the benefits of deep breathing?

Deep breathing using the full lung capacity allows us to get into the deep low lobes of the lungs. By breathing mainly into the upper chest, we can overuse the accessory muscles around the neck and this can create tension. Breathing with control can help facilitate movement without tension. By trying to use our full lung capacity, we allow more oxygen into our body so more blood can be purified and more energy passed around the body.

How do you use the full lung capacity?

This is not something we can be conscious of doing all day every day but it is something we can practice when we come to yoga. Or at some point during the day, find a still point and take a few deep, long breaths. The focus should be to expand the ribcage, belly and chest to use the full lung capacity. Ensuring the breath is long and slow.

What can restrict us?

There are a number of things that can restrict full deep

breathing, of course, kyphosis i.e., the upper back flexes forward will create a limitation in the expansion of the ribcage and of course will make deep breathing more challenging. Tight muscles around the ribcage will limit how much we can expand the ribcage laterally and posteriorly. Most of the time when we inhale in yoga, it helps to promote spinal extension so if a person's natural posture is more kyphotic, this will make it more challenging but all the more reason to help try to change this. Have you ever wondered why the half-moon pose is so early on in the hot series? It opens the lateral sides of the body in particular the thoracic spine area. Thus, creating more mobility and space, which helps with breathing.

Benefits of deep breathing

Simply we take more oxygen in we have more fresh oxygen to go into the blood, which can help send oxygenated blood to the muscles to help them to work more efficiently. It also helps to slow the heart rate, which in turn will calm the nervous system.

You may have heard of 'fight-or-flight mode'. This is when the sympathetic nervous system responds to an event or situation that might cause stress or fear, with a sudden release of hormones the body will become tense and the breathing will become shallow. Palms might get sweaty, your heart beats faster and your breathing is faster.

Imagine if a tiger was running at you this would trigger the fight-or-flight response and notice what we tend to do with our body we close down. This is normal but the effect of this closing down of the body makes it harder for us to breathe deeply. I know what you're thinking: if a tiger is running at me I am not going to stand there and focus on breathing deep. But this very same siltation can occur when we public speak or we are on an aeroplane. Certainly, in the public speaking situation, we don't need to fear death, so this is when we can use breathing to help control how we feel.

Notice on the opposite end of the scale when you are having a massage or meditating you feel totally calm and your breathing is slow and relaxed. You feel calm your heart beats at a regular or slightly slower pace. In this state is much easier for us to think clearer and make a more informed decision. It can often happen when I first started teaching we will get very nervous before teaching and as much as I can say don't worry you will. Honestly, it's a good thing it means you care about what you are about to do so it's a good sign. But knowing how we can control our heart and feelings using our breath my advice would be to try to take a few deep breaths before class to help calm the nervous system ever so slightly.

So, what type of breathing techniques should we teach in our classes and how difficult is it. The first you need to consider is what is the goal, do you want to heat the body or cool the body down? Do you want to energise the students or calm them down? Is it good to start class with a breathing exercise or finish, like I say it depends on your goals. So let's look at some options of simple techniques you can teach your students.

Examples of breathing exercises

The first is the simplest it's just about becoming aware of your breath. Taking time to focus your attention on your breathing. Becoming aware of inhaling and exhaling. Taking time to become still is great for generally calming down the nervous system. It's a great way to start a yoga class especially if people have rushed from a busy day at the office. By taking a minute or two to centre yourself and prepare for practice is a great way to start class. By focusing on the breath, we can slow down the heart and mind if the perfect way to start your yoga practice.

How it's done:

- Sit long and tall in a comfortable seated position, roll your shoulders down a back, reach the crown of the head up to the ceiling soften your face and gently close your eyes.
- Become aware of your body here this is now the time for you, be aware of any tension or tightness in the body and send your breath to that area.
- Take a long slow deep inhale, and a long slow deep exhale. Inhaling through the nose and exhaling through the nose.
- With every breath, try to deepen the inhale and lengthen the exhale.
- Feel the ribs, chest and belly expand as you inhale and as you exhale the belly chest and ribs relax and soften.
- Feel your heart begin to slow as your breath deepens. Keep your mind focused on your breath.

Another simple option would be to have students lie down on the mat and have them count their breaths for one minute. Complete the exercise again and ask them if they can half the number. Ideally, you would take only three long slow breaths in one minute. Calming the nervous system, the mind and slowing the heart. Our minds get so distracted it's hard to just focus on breathing sometimes but it's very beneficial for our well-being.

Kapalbhati – mouth or nose version (breath of fire)

There are two versions of this breathing, one with the mouth open and one with the mouth closed. One is more cooling and one is more warming. The cooling variation you may have practised in a hot yoga class. This is traditionally done at the end of class to help cool the body down. Kapalbhati is not only a breathing exercise but also a cleansing exercise as it helps to clear out the lungs and helps to strengthen the abs. it also increases the oxygen supply, which helps the brain function.

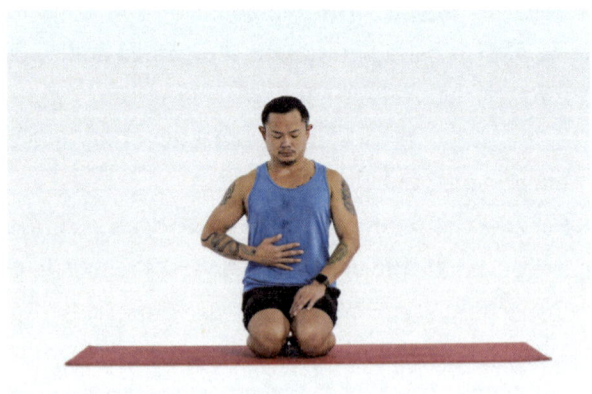

Breathing

How it's done:

- Find a comfortable seated position either crossed-legged or kneeling. (easy pose or hero pose)
- Hands resting on your knees. Sit long and tall with a straight spine.
- Don't worry about the inhale as this will happen automatically.
- Inhale through the nose as you exhale contract your low abs and pull the belly into the spine forcing the air out of your mouth.
- You can do this for 10 reps anything up to one minute.
- Once you finish, take a long inhale and deep exhale.

The variation of exhaling through the mouth is focused on cooling the body down and is generally done at the end of class. If you keep your mouth closed and exhale through the nose, this is more of a warming practice and so is good to do at the start of class. You may have done this type of breathing in a hot yoga class. There are many benefits including detoxing the lungs, strengthening the abs, increasing oxygen in the body and calming the nervous system.

Inhale and exhale for four counts

This is more of a calming breathing exercise and it's nice to do at the end of class. This breathing will help return breathing to a calm normal pattern, i.e., breathing like normal but with a calmness about you. This is a simple and great exercise to do at any point when you feel under pressure or stressed.

- Find a comfortable seated position either cross-legged or kneeling. (easy pose or hero pose)
- Hands resting on your knees. Sit long and tall with a straight spine.
- Inhale for 1, 2, 3, 4…Pause.
- Exhale 4, 3, 2, 1, Pause.
- Again Inhale for 1, 2, 3, 4…Pause.
- Exhale 4, 3, 2, 1, Pause.

Keep breathing like this long and slow and with every exhale see if you lengthen the exhale a little longer…

- Inhale for 1, 2, 3, 4…Pause.
- Exhale 5, 4, 3, 2, 1, Pause.

The Inhale slightly increases your heart rate, whereas the exhale slows your heart down so by lengthening your exhale you allow the body to relax more and decrease tension. Each time you practise maybe increase the length of the exhale until eventually you exhale for eight and inhale for four.

Alternate nostril breathing

There are many benefits to alternate nostril breathing. Often we tend to favour one side of the body or one lung due to muscle tightness so this is a great exercise to help rebalance the body. It can help reduce stress, increase lung function and increase respiratory endurance. Depending on what nostril you inhale can also determine if you are calming the body, left nostril or more energised right nostril. By breathing into the left first can direct oxygen to the right hemisphere of the brain and which turns on the parasympathetic system. If you breathe into the right first, it helps to increase energy within the body.

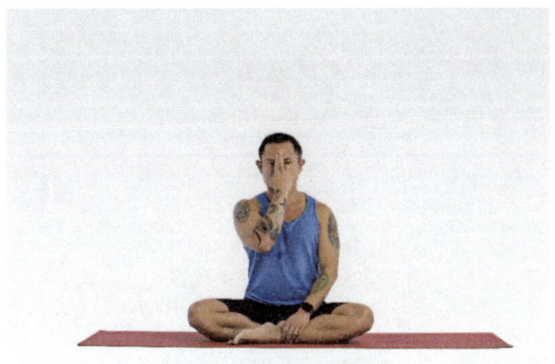

Breathing

There are many versions of alternative nostril breathing. This version is a simple variation here. I have chosen to start with the right side but you can start with the left.

- Find a comfortable seated position sit long and tall. Use a block if you need to.
- Relax the left hand onto your leg and lift the right palm in front of your face.
- First and second finger on your forehead, thumb on your right nostril and ring finger on the left.
- Close your left nostril and inhale through the right.
- Close both nostrils and pause.
- Keep the right nostril closed and open the left and exhale through the left.
- Inhale through the left nostril, close both nostrils and pause.

- Open the right and exhale through the right.
- Continue this through 10–15 cycles.

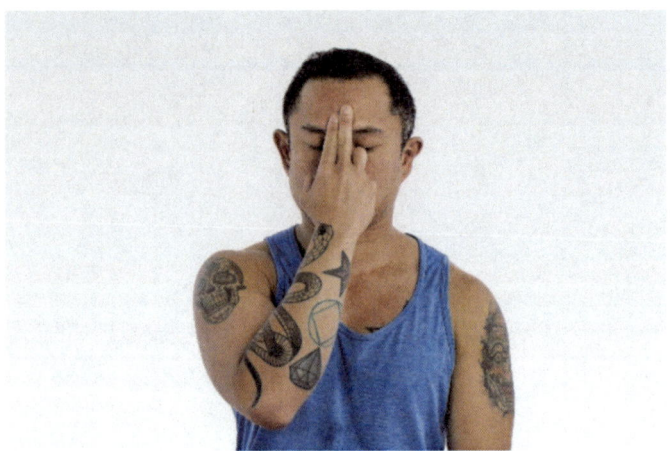

Close up

Chapter 12
Meditation

Do you need to teach meditation in class is a question you need to ask yourself? It's really a personal choice some people like to teach it and some people don't. If you are not comfortable teaching something, then you don't have to teach it. Not everyone teaches the same yoga class and so omitting meditation if that's your preference is okay. You can simply have people lie down in savasana and relax in silence at the end of class. There are no rules that a yoga class must have meditation at any point during the class it is simply a personal choice.

Benefits of meditation

- Reduce stress
- Controls anxiety
- Self-awareness
- Better concentration
- Inner peace

Mediation does not need to look like some formal part of the class it can be simply bringing your attention to your breath, creating stillness or even a focused mediation. Simply taking some time to stop during a busy day has many benefits.

How to teach meditation

This is not generally something that is taught during a teacher-training course I think, because it's assumed it's easy. But if you have never done it before it can be a challenge. It's very easy to buy a book with meditations or Yoga Nidra readings but often what is missing is the set-up of meditation and how to finish and end the class. So I have included them here in case you need them. Mediation can be done seated or in a supine position. I have always found that supine works better, as people are less likely to fidget; they are more likely to fall asleep though. The tone of voice is important when teaching meditation, so find your 'spa' voice, soften the tone, decrease the volume lengthen the words and make it slow and deliberate.

Examples of mediation – Prep, finisher and samples

Prep 1

Lie down on your back and close your eyes. Relax all the muscles in your body from the crown of the head to the tips of your toes. (Pause) Feel your shoulders broaden and sink down into the mat, and allow your feet to flop out to the sides.

Relax your forehead and eyebrows. Allow the hips to release and allow the legs and arms to relax. Let your whole body melt down into the mat. (Pause) Allow your breath to deepen and feel your heart begin to slow down as you sink deeper. With every breath, you sink deeper and deeper into relaxation. (Pause) Today we will take a short journey to… (Name the story here i.e., golden bay)

Prep 2

Lie down on your back and close your eyes. Allow your whole body to sink into the mat. Become aware of your arms, take a deep inhale breath into your arms, tense all the muscles in your arms and exhale let it go. Become aware of your legs, take a deep inhale, breathe into your legs, tense all the muscles in your legs and exhale and let it go. Become aware of your face, take a deep inhale breath into your face, tense all the muscles in your face and exhale and let it go. Become aware of your whole body, tense all the muscles in the whole body, breathe into the tension and exhale and let it go. (Pause). Allow your body to melt and sink into the mat, let the mat support your body as you begin your relaxation. Today we will take a short journey to… (Name the story here i.e., golden bay)

Prep 3

Allow your body to begin to relax from the crown of the head to the tips of your toes. Allow your body to sink into your mat, and allow your mat to support your body whilst you relax. (Pause) Feel your breath begin to deepen, allow your eyes to sink into pools or darkness and completely let go. Just focus on feeling the belly rise as you inhale, pause, and belly fall as you exhale. Today we will take a short journey to… (Name the story here i.e., golden bay)

Once you finish the story, give students a couple of minutes of silence and then finish the mediation with what I call the finisher.

Finisher

Begin to deepen your breath, become aware of the body again and be aware of your body here lying on your mat. (Pause) Notice how it feels now, stronger yet lighter energised yet relaxed. (Pause) Begin to wiggle your fingers and toes, bringing some life back to your body. Take the arms overhead and give yourself a full body stretch, stretch both arms and legs. Release the arms down by your side, hugs the knees into the chest, rock over to the right side, make a pillow with your hands and rest here. (Pause) Whenever you are ready come up to a comfortable seated position. Facing the front with your eyes closed. Sit long and tall slide your shoulders down and back. Inhale, reach the arms overhead palms together in a prayer position, exhale, hands to your heart, bow your head and blink your eyes open, and lift your head looking forward.

See the options below for something you can then say. It needs to resonate with you so choose one that works for you or use one of your own.

"Thank you for coming to class."

"Namaste."

"Thanks for sharing your practice with me today."

"Thank yourself for your effort in your practice today."

"Have a good day and come back soon."

Below are some examples of meditations you don't need to use but I have included them so you have some options you can use if you feel that it's suitable.

Golden Bay

Today we will take a short journey to the golden bay. It is almost sunset on a beautiful summer evening, and you decide to take a stroll on the beach. You walk along the beach, it is a beautiful evening you can feel the warmth of the golden sand under your feet, and the energy of the sun shines on your face. (Pause) As you stroll further up the beach the tide draws in and out, every now and then as the tide draws in you feel the fresh cool ocean between your toes.

As you continue walking, you look down and see the stones and shells that are around on the beach. There are lots of shapes and sizes, you stop to take a closer look, you notice that one catches your eye, and you feel yourself drawn to this one. It's a perfectly round stone, pure marble white in colour, it's not very big yet stands out amongst them all. (Pause) You reach down and pick it up, as you hold it in your hand, it feels as smooth as silk. Although it's white in colour as you turn the stone, you can see light shades of other colours within the stone. Keep turning the stone until you find a colour you are drawn to, which one stands outs and draws you in. There is no one around so you decide to take the stone and walk further up the beach to golden bay.

The golden bay is deserted, you sit down on the sand and enjoy the peace. Holding the stone in your hand you close your eyes and feel the light breeze from the ocean and the warmth of the sun. You hold the stone tight in your hand; you begin to drift into a deeper, relaxed state. Thoughts of the day pass through your mind, but you don't hold on to any you just observe.

You notice that the stone begins to warm as it sits tightly in your hand. Feel the purity in the stone and allow the stone to take away all the worries of the day. You begin to drift deeper and as you drift; you start to feel light throughout your body as your worries leave your body. (Pause) Your whole body feels lighter and you notice there is more space within your body. As you focus on sending your worries to the stone, you feel it begin to warm a little more. Your body is light it feels energised and your mind feels clearer with more space. (Pause for a minute or two)

You become aware of yourself still sitting on the golden sand; you begin to gently open your eyes you notice that the sun is a little lower and more orange. You are still holding the stone and you notice the heat within it and the lightness around you. You get up and walk to the ocean shore, you no longer need the stone it's done all it needed to do. You decide to throw the stone into the ocean to wash away all the worries from today. The stone lands with two hops and a plop deep into the ocean and you feel lighter and free. You walk back down the beach with calmness and clarity that you are brighter and there is an extra spring in your step. (Pause) With the lightness and calmness around your body begin to deepen your breath. Small gentle movements start to wake the body up once more feeling that lightness and calmness around you.

Behind the Falls

It's a frosty dark morning and you are walking in the park. In the middle of the park is a large open lake, you decide to head for the lake to see the sunrise. Once you get nearer to the lake, you notice it's a little misty, so chances are you won't get to see the sunrise this morning. You walk around the outside of the lake, there are dog walkers walking their dogs, and people running, and biking. You head into the trees it feels cooler here, as you head in deeper you can hear the sounds of running water and you decide to head in the direction of the water sound, as you get closer the rushing water sound gets louder, much louder. (Pause)

Finally, you make it into a clearing and you see in front of you a waterfall, it's beautifully surrounded by trees and green plants, and the water cascades down the side of the hill to a small stream. You take a moment to feel the energy from the water although the sound of the water is rather loud you enjoy listening to it.

You stand for a moment and close your eyes to feel the energy, the coolness in the air brushing over your face. You begin to imagine what it would be like standing under this waterfall, the cool breeze in the air you begin to smile and enjoy this moment of being here with such a beautiful waterfall. After a few moments, you open your eyes and walk around to one side of the waterfall and you notice a small door. The door is a small wooden door, surrounded by bushes and trees; you could almost miss it if you did not look close enough.

You wonder where does this door leads to, so you get closer to the door. You notice a small handle, it's a little rusty but you reach out and turn the handle, with one simple click the door opens. You take a step forward and look in, you see some stairs leading down, so you decide to investigate further. (Pause) As you make your way down the stairs you feel the coolness within. With every step, you take the sound of the rushing water gets even louder and the air gets cooler.

Finally, you reach the bottom and you find yourself behind the waterfall. The water is cascading down right in front of your eyes. The air is cool but still, you observe the way the water falls down like a big sheet of glass in front of you. You close your eyes once again and listen to the sounds around you. The sound of the water takes you deeper into a relaxed state and you find your mind drifts off. You imagine yourself standing directly under the waterfall. You can feel the cool fresh water rushing over your body, how cool and energised it makes you feel. You feel as if your body is being soaked in life force and healing energy. Washing away all that you don't need, all the negative thoughts all the pain and all the concerns just washes away as the water flows. You tip your head back and enjoy every moment.

(Pause for a minute or two)

You feel revitalised, energised and relaxed. You feel as if your whole body is drenched in calming energy. Your mind drifts back once again to where you are and you find yourself behind the waterfall. You open your eyes and through the curtain of water you can see the sun is fully up, a new day has begun. It's time to leave, you walk back up the stairs towards the wooden door. With each step you take, you feel ready for what the rest of the day has to offer. You reach the top, open the door and head back towards the lake. You leave the lakeside and return to the entrance of the park. In your mind, knowing the secret door to the back of the waterfall will be there any time you need to visit. Anytime you feel the need for some energy.

The Rocking Chair

One day you are out for a stroll when it begins to rain light at first but it starts to get heavier. You stand undercover outside a shop to shelter from the rain, you look into the window and notice it's a second-hand store, as you look through the window and see some interesting items and decide to go in. You walk through the entrance glancing at various items such as chairs, lamps, desks and antique trinkets.

As you browse through the store, the owner comes over to talk to you. He is an older gentleman with glasses that sit on the perch of his nose; he is wearing light casual trousers and a white shirt. "Is there anything I can assist you with?" he says.

"No, I am just browsing thank you," you say.

"No problem, just ask if you need any help?" he says as he wanders off to help another customer who is looking at some lamps.

You walk further down to the back of the shop, it seems endless, how could such a small fronted shop be so large inside. As you turn a corner you notice a rocking chair, it's made of wood and embossed with a logo at the top with some writing. (Pause) You look closer and it says, "Journey to peace," you have a quick look around and no one appears to be in this part of the shop so you decide to sit down on the chair. It's very comfortable, it seems to mould around your body, you gently rock back and forth and think how wonderful it would be to own such a beautiful chair. As you rock a little more you close your eyes and imagine you are on your journey to peace. You wonder what peace looks like, what it feels like, is there a bright white light. With every rock forward and back, you drift deeper. You wonder if there is a garden full of flowers or a long sandy beach. On this journey, there is everything you so desire, is it a room full of scented candles (pause) or a garden of flowers (pause) or a beautiful sunset or simply inner peace. What you notice is the silence, a silence of the mind, (pause) stillness in the body (pause). You feel a sense of calmness flood through your body from the crown of your head to the tips of your toes. A feeling you have not felt for a while. You take some time to enjoy this stillness gently rocking back and forth.

(Pause for a minute or two)

After a while, you hear some voices in the background, and you begin to bring your mind back into your body. You become aware of your senses and aware of where you are. You open your eyes and get up from the chair, you notice you feel more peaceful, more relaxed and with a clearer mind. You walk to the front of the store and thank the kind owner, he says it's no problem please come again anytime soon.

As you walk out of the store, you see the rain has stopped and the sun is shining bright in the sky, you know today is going to be a good day.

The orchard

It's a summer's day and you find yourself walking through the meadow. The sun is shining brightly; butterflies are floating around as you walk through a meadow of wildflowers. Poppies, sunflowers, pansies and many varieties of flowers create a sea of colour in front of your eyes. As you walk further through the meadow, you finally reach a gate, it's an old gate which has a rusty lock, you can't open the lock the rust prevents the lock from being opened. You see in the distance there is a path intrigued by what lies beyond the path you decide to climb over the gate.

You climb over the gate and walk further on, as you reach the other side you see the path more clearly, you walk towards the path. As you get closer, you can see the path separates two parts of the meadow, wildflowers are on either side. There is a path going to the left and also the right. (Pause)

The path to the left appears clear it looks like it's an easy walk with beautiful flowers on each side and the sunlight dappling down through the trees. The opposite way seems to be more overgrown with weeds and the trees hang over the path, blocking the sunlight. Your instinct says to take the left path no need to take the right one that seems to be more challenging. Whilst you contemplate which path to take you to notice a white butterfly, it seems unusual in colour, as all the ones you saw earlier were brightly coloured. It flies around and eventually flies off down the right path. Is it a sign that you should take the right path? Something now tells you that you should take the right path, which appears more complicated.

You're not in a hurry, you have plenty of time so you decide to take the right path; the grass is long, it's full of weeds and overgrown plants; it does not feel as beautiful as you imagine the other path to be. As you walk further, the vegetation is denser and heavier it feels damp and cold. You can't see the sunlight anymore there is too much vegetation blocking the light, and each step becomes a little more difficult. With sharp branches blocking the way, you wonder why you decided to come this way. As you continue to plod on, you notice the white butterfly again. Something tells you that although it's hard, it's the right way to go.

A walk further towards the end of the path you notice another gate, this one is a large wooden gate it's a beautiful gate with a brass lock that shines in the sunshine. The gate includes a sign that says, "Fruits of your labour," you wonder why such a sign would be here so you open the gate and wander through. As you close the gate, you march through the overgrown bushes it's a hard slog but you keep going. You do begin to wonder why you chose this path, it's difficult with so many overgrown plants and bushes and the ground you walk on is not easy terrain either.

Eventually, you find a clearing and you find yourself in an orchard of apple trees, as far as the eye can see there are apple trees. Tall trees with long thin trunks, full of green and red delights hanging from the branches shining bright in the sunshine. The apples hang freely bobbing around in the gentle breeze. (Pause) You decide to walk further past trees with, green apples, and bright red apples, some are small and some are very large. As the wind blows you can smell the scent of apples. You walk further towards the shaded area and as you pass one of the green trees, a perfectly round green apple falls to the ground. You bend down and pick it up. You look around and there is no one to be seen, so you sit down and decide to eat the apple. You take a bite of the apple, it's firm and crisp with a delicious sweetness. Never have you tasted such a delicious apple before. You close your eyes to fully experience the deliciousness of the apple. It reminds you of when you were young, wild and free. It reminds you of playful times when there was no care in the world. As you sit here you realise there is nothing to worry about, nothing to be concerned about simply enjoy the freshness of the apple. You breathe deep and you can smell the scent of fresh apples, you feel the cool breeze on your face and you feel good. (Pause)

The sun starts to fade and you realise it's time to return back to the meadow. You open your eyes, with the feeling of freshness and lightness you walk back to the gate and return to the meadow.

Chapter 13
Teaching Online

How to teach online

The new normal, not even sure what that means but for sure teaching will not be the same again at least for a while. During a number of lockdowns during covid, teachers have taken their classes online, which is a great option to keep connected to students during lockdown times. But like anything, there is a good way to do it and an okay way. So if you have never taught online before, then how do you know what to do and how different it is?

Surely you just stick your phone camera on and off you go. Of course, you can do just that but in order to make it easy for clients to sign up, you want to make it good. Lots of clients don't like to train online they prefer to come to the studio so motivating people is a job in itself. So first ask do you want to run online classes? If you do, then what equipment do you need? These days it does not need to be fancy most computers and phones have pretty good cameras in them. You need to think about how you will deliver the class, i.e., will you simply go live and students follow you or do you want it interactive where you can see students therefore zoom might be a better option.

Of course, it depends on your situation but do you charge or is it free? This is a hard one as there are so much free online these days. However, if you have a studio or a group of students who love you and your classes, then they might be willing to pay something to join but you can't charge the same as a regular group class. So consider if you have the right equipment or if you need to invest in something new. I used my MacBook computer and Air pods and the sound and visual was pretty good.

Camera position

It's important you have a good camera position, it needs to be high up and set in a horizontal position. You will also be surprised how far the camera needs to be away from you. You need to see the full length of the mat and the full length of your body standing. The camera should point down slightly so you can see the full yoga mat.

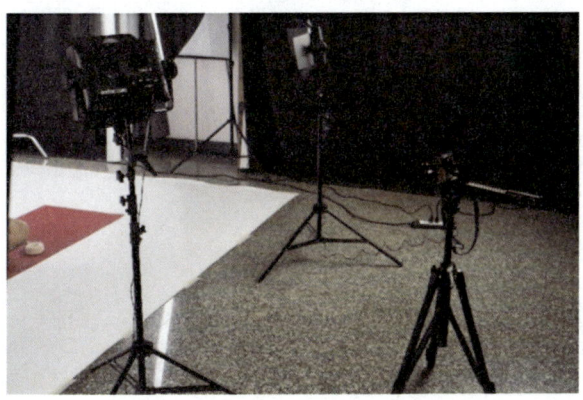

You can see the camera behind the lights in order to ensure there is plenty of light. The set-up here is more for closer shots you would need to move the camera or yoga mat back more for full-body shots.

Lighting

It's very important that you can be seen clearly. Windows should be behind the camera otherwise the lighting looks too dark. If you can also have an extra spotlight so that you can be seen clearly. Try to move furniture and distractions out of the way so you have enough space for your mat. If people know you are running classes online from home, so it's okay to see some furniture but make it look reasonably tidy.

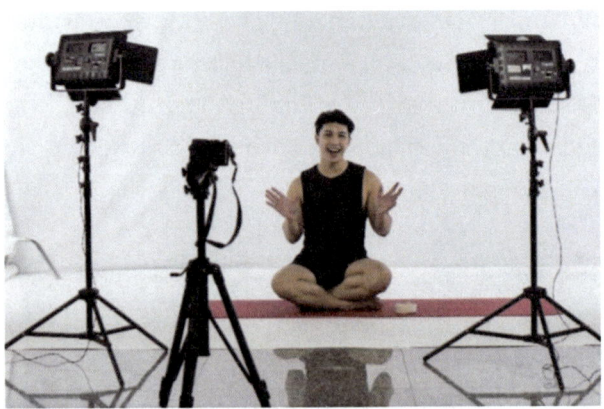

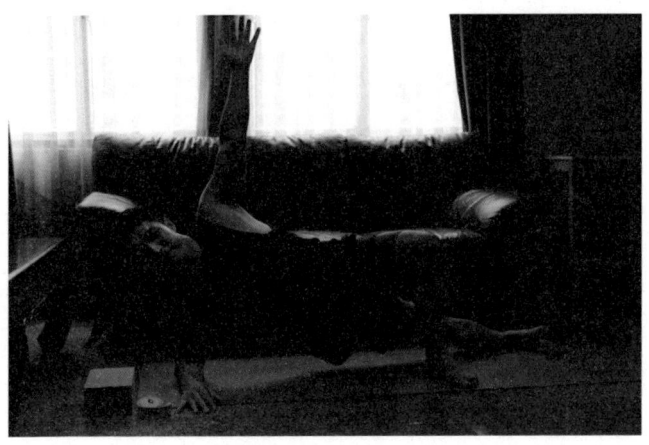

Wrong Camera Position

You can see the scene is well lit and although this is a more professional set-up with the white screen, it's more to give you an idea of what you can do. White background with bounce light back so will make it appear. You don't need professional equipment like this but with two good lights, it can make all the difference.

Audio

Always use a microphone, even if it's ear pods you will be far from the camera and you need to be heard clearly. I personally found the apple Air pods worked great. You will be moving around and sometimes you may need to demonstrate a little bit so you need to hear very clearly. Make sure you have a good internet connection and there are no other things around that will distract you i.e., kids, dogs, or a phone ringing. I know that sometimes these things can't be helped but try to minimise distractions as much as possible. Always test all of this before class starts with a friend or someone online. Make sure you can be seen and heard. There is nothing worse than having technical issues right before you are about to start class.

Zoom is a great option as you are able to see students and give them verbal corrections. If you do use Zoom, ensure that all students are set to mute once the class starts so that no noise from their end can be heard either.

Dialogue

This is one of the most important tools in your toolkit. As you are not able to physically adjust students your instructions need to be super clear and detailed. You want students to practice and not keep coming up to the camera and looking at what you are doing. As the class is starting up and people join, you might want to chitchat a bit, this gives everyone a chance to join and then the class can start together. People sometimes struggle with the technology aspect so you can always open the Zoom room a few minutes early and let people know. If someone does join late, you might find that you need to repeat instructions. The first time they do it, it might be a bit messy if they are not familiar with technology but they will get used to it. What is also nice touch is to send detailed instructions on how they can set up Zoom prior to the class. I've found the best way is to chitchat a bit at first, "Hi, how are you, Lisa," etc. "Okay, let's start in two minutes," wait for everyone to be there or the majority and then start.

Props

If you need props, tell them ahead of time or tell them during the chitchat so they have time to collect what they need. You also need to consider if you use props that people might not have them so maybe instead of a block, it's a cushion or a water bottle instead of a dumbbell. It needs to be things they can find in their home. Most people have a bottle of water, a cushion or a towel so it's easy to access them.

Demonstration

You will probably need to demonstrate more than normal but remember you only need to demo the pose once and don't need to do both sides. Please also note that you will need to mirror the students if you are face on, i.e., say left leg you do right. Otherwise, students will get confused. However when sideways you can do the same side. This makes it less confusing for students and they can copy you even if they can't hear you too well.

Sequence

The one thing about teaching online is to teach simple poses and ones you know students can do without requiring an adjustment. There is no point teaching some fancy arm balances if most can't do it because you are not able to help them. If you teach things they know, then it's easy to follow along, warrior 2 most people know but some fancy poses might not work as it takes too much explanation and maybe you need to demonstrate too much and you could lose interest from students. Simple fun and flowing is all you need. You still make students work hard but holding poses longer like warrior 2 or boat. If people know it's not going to be too difficult, they are more likely to join. It's hard enough to get people to join online classes as it is. Make clear the style of class you are offering if it sounds difficult it could put people off.

Music

It's nice to include music but make sure it does not take over your voice so it's more background music. The most important part is that you can be heard so make that priority. I personally did not include music during class as I did not want to distract from my voice but I would use it at the end for final relaxation.

Interaction with students

This is very important as we are not able to connect with them in person and it helps to make them feel part of a group whilst students are holding a pose come up to the camera and have a look and maybe comment, "Lisa, turn your back toes in," "Mike, great job." This is why you don't need to demo both sides once they did one side they know roughly what is happening so that's when you can connect with people. Also, take some time after class to have quick chitchat and see how everyone feels. Saying students' names can really make them feel like the experience was good and they are not just following some random YouTube video of someone they don't know. That's the personal touch and that's why they paid to join your class.

Mistakes made by most teachers

The main areas in which teachers make mistakes when teaching online concern audio and visual aspects. Most of the time they don't have a microphone and therefore can't always be heard clearly. This of course is made worse when the teacher does the poses with the students and then has their heads in their legs so it's even more muffled.

The other big mistake is lighting, most people tend to focus so much on making the view look good they often have bad lighting like below. The window should always be behind the camera unless you have lots of additional lights. I don't mean table lamps from the bedroom I mean proper lights for a video that can be facing towards yourself.

Style of yoga classes you can teach online

Keep it simple, when you don't have any physical contact with the students, you are relying on that they can hear and understand you through the camera. The Internet can sometimes not be reliable and you don't want students to have to keep looking at the screen so it's best to do things you know they can understand and do. Most of the time they simply just want to keep moving until they are able to attend a class at the studio again. With the rise of COVID, more and more people will be looking to have classes online, especially those that feel more vulnerable so if you start with a client online and it could be their first time ever doing yoga. So, prepare a simple sequence which you can adjust if need be. Familiarity is important so do things that make people feel good and they will continue to train with you.

Conclusion

Teaching yoga is not easy. It is physically exhausting and emotionally draining, but it's also incredibly rewarding. So much of what we do each day and in each class has such a positive effect on people. I'm grateful to be able to share that gift with so many people in so many different countries. My goal with this book was to share all that I've learned in the hopes that it helps someone become a better teacher. What is it that you want to achieve? It might simply be to become a good yoga teacher, maybe open a great studio, or perhaps one day have your own training course. Whatever your personal goals are, you must believe in them, imagine them, and work hard.

I'd like to finish with a story of a student in one of my training courses; she was a lady who worked in the corporate business, she was in her 50s and came along to the course because her sister dragged her along. She loved yoga in terms of practice but was not sure if she wanted to become a teacher. Every time she stood up to teach she would lose her words, she could not speak, she could not even think of what the next pose was, yet her presence was electric, I could feel something about her that I knew she would be a great teacher. It took a whole month of hard work and even, in the end, I thought she would never make it. If someone is likely to fail, it was always my job to assess his or her exam, so here I was for the final exam of this very lady. The full class is 90 minutes and the teaching is split between two people so they teach for 45 minutes each. To give more of a group class feel they have anything from 6–8 students in class, who are of course also teacher trainees too.

The grouping is always done by lucky dip and interesting enough one of the 'students' in the class was her sister. Even as I write these words, I get goose bumps and it makes me smile ear to ear. I observed all of her class and write down copious notes to pass on to her after class; I could not believe what I was seeing. Something had changed overnight and she was a different person. I tell people on my course I can teach you the words and the poses and how to structure a class but the passion comes from within, her passion was shining bright this day. As I gave her my feedback, I had tears rolling down my cheeks I was so delighted and amazed at what I was seeing. Her sister was stuck for words, which was unusual for her. This is why I do this job, it's hard work, especially for teacher training courses, but to be part of a journey like this is magic that you could not conjure up with a wand.

I hope that this book brings some magic into your life and I hope that you continue to learn and be ever grateful for this amazing job that we have.

Namaste.